DATE

Alcohol and the Identification of Alcoholics

A Handbook for Professionals

BY

H.G. Giles

AND

B.M. Kapur
Addiction Research Foundation
and the
University of Toronto

Lexington Books

D.C. Heath and Company/Lexington, Massachusetts/Toronto

Managing Editor: S. Sandrin

The views expressed and positions taken in this book are those of
the authors and do not necessarily represent the views or positions
of the Addiction Research Foundation.

Library of Congress Cataloging-in-Publication Data

Giles, H.G. (H. Gwynne)
    Alcohol and the identification of alcoholics in legal proceedings
by H.G. Giles, B.M. Kapur.
    p. cm.
    Includes index.
    ISBN 0-669-24923-8
    1. Alcohol—Physiological effect. 2. Blood alcohol—Analysis.
3. Alcoholics—Identification. 4. Alcoholics—Legal status, laws,
etc.—United States. I. Kapur, B.M. (Bhushan M.) II. Title.
QP801.A3G55   1991
616.86′1—dc20
                                                    90-42275
                                                    CIP

Published simultaneously in Canada
Printed in the United States of America
International Standard Book Number: 0-669-24923-8
Library of Congress Catalog Card Number: 90-42275

The paper used in this publication meets the minimum
requirements of American National Standard for Information
Sciences—Permanence of Paper for Printed Library Materials,
ANSI Z39.48-1984.

Year and number of this printing:
91 92 93 94 8 7 6 5 4 3 2 1

Contents

Preface   ix

Acknowledgments   xi

1. Basics   1
    Names   1
    Origin   1
    Characteristics   2
    Uses   2
    Units of Concentration   2
    Concentration of Alcoholic Beverages   3
    Conversion of Units   4
    Volume of a Drink   4
    The Weight of Pure Alcohol in a Drink   6
    Alcohol: A Hidden Ingredient   7

2. How Does Alcohol Get into the Body and Where
    Does It Go?   9
    Factors that influence absorption   10
    The "Last Gulp" Defense   12
    Distribution of Alcohol into Body Fluids   12
    Body Water   12
    Estimating the Maximum Concentration in Body Water   14
    Blood   14

Blood Plasma   14

Blood Serum   15

Other Liquids   15

Erroneous Reporting of "Blood" Alcohol Concentration   16

Breath   16

Units of Concentration   17

Estimating the Maximum Blood Alcohol
Concentration (BAC)   18

Breast Milk   18

Estimating the Minimum Alcohol Ingested   19

Attempts to Reduce Alcohol Concentration by
Drinking Water   20

Attempts to Reduce Alcohol Concentration by Sweating   20

Blood Transfusions and Blood Loss   20

3.   What Happens to Alcohol in the Body?   23

Rule of Thumb for "Safe" Alcohol Consumption   23

Breakdown of the Rule of Thumb   24

Metabolic Tolerance   24

Traumatic Injuries   25

Nutritional Factors That Affect Alcohol Metabolism   26

What is a Flusher?   26

What Is Endogenous Alcohol?   26

Concentration Versus Time Profile   27

Problems with Back-Calculations   28

When Does the Concentration Reach Its Peak?   29

How Curved Is the Straight-Line Portion of the Curve?   30

More on the Dreaded Back-Calculations   31

Excretion of Alcohol   34

4.   Toxic Effects of Alcohol   35

Contents

Short-term Toxicity   35
Long-term toxicity   39
Reversibility of Toxic Effects   44

5.   Effect of Alcohol on Other Substances and Vice Versa   45
Effect of Alcohol on Other Substances   45
Effect of Other Substances on Alcohol   47

6.   Women and Alcohol   51
Body Size   51
Total Body Water   51
Oral Contraceptives and Alcohol   53
Menstrual Cycle   53
Short-term Toxicity   54
Long-term Toxicity   54
Breast Feeding   54

7.   Analysis of Alcohol   55
Blood Samples   55
Preservation of Liquid Samples   56
Analysis of Alcohol in Liquids   57
Analysis of Alcohol in Breath   58
Errors in Instrumental Analysis Alone   59
Samples Obtained after Death   61
Other Errors   62
Forensic Transposition of Concentrations   62
Breath Analysis   64
Urine Analysis   70
Recommendations for Reform: Statutory Definition for All Body Fluids   73

8.   Traffic Accidents   77
Alcohol and the Risk of a Traffic Accident   77

The RISK Computer Program   78
The "Morning After" and Driving   80

9. Program for Estimating Blood and Breath Alcohol
    Concentrations (BBAC)   81
    Using BBAC: An Example   81
    General Remarks   86
    Brand Name Tables   88

10. Identification of Alcoholics in Legal Proceedings   93
    The Importance of Identifying an Alcoholic   93
    "It Takes One to Know One" . . . Or Does It?   94
    The General Method   94
    What Approaches Are Impractical?   94
    What Is an Alcoholic?   95
    Is You Is or Is You Ain't . . . an Alcoholic?   98
    What Are the Tests Going to Tell?   100
    Four Meanings of "Outside the Normal Range"   100

11. Tests for Alcoholism   103
    Tests Based on Tolerance   103
    Other Tests Based upon the Direct Measurement
    of Alcohol   106
    Questionnaires and Appearance   107
    Death Certificates   112
    Frequency of Changing Jobs   113
    Other Blood Tests for Alcoholism   113
    ID: Computer Program for the Identification of Alcohol
    Abuse/Dependence   115

12. Court-Ordered Treatment of Alcoholism   117
    Distinguishing Alcohol Abuse and Alcohol Dependence   118
    The Category Determines the Treatment   118
    Assessment of the Results of Treatment   119

Appendix 1: Conversion Tables   121

Appendix 2: Glasgow Coma Scale   123

A Note on the Companion Computer Programs   125

Index   129

About the Authors   132

Accurate
Perspective

Preface

T he object of this book is to make scientific work on alcohol
and alcoholism available to nonscientists.

There are millions of people throughout the world who respon-
sibly enjoy consuming alcoholic beverages. There are others,
though, whose drinking generates serious problems.

In every industrialized country, in every year, there are hundreds of thousands of people charged with alcohol-related offenses.
This problem is ten times larger than offenses related to other
drugs. Alcohol consumption is also a major factor in civil cases,
most obviously those involving torts, divorce, employment, and the
care of young children. Alcohol consumption and alcoholism can
also be issues in many other areas that involve reliability, capacity,
or health.

This book is intended to provide an adequate basis of knowledge for the nonscientist to use when the occasion demands, and
also to allow him to recognize those times when an expert or a
specialist source needs to be consulted. Many books, periodicals,
and even institutions are dedicated to the toxic effects of alcohol,
but in this book we cover much of the subject in one chapter. Still,
the information given is sufficient for the purposes of the book,
and we give a little more to keep alive the interest of the reader
and the academic pretenses of the authors.

The last chapters of the book cover the identification of alcoholics. This field is somewhat new, and the principles are still being
developed. It is presented here so that it may be used in legal proceedings where there are procedures in place to safeguard individual rights. The area is being developed by research scientists pri-

marily to help in the medical treatment of patients. It is not being developed to allow unfair discrimination against alcoholics, so we do not answer inquiries from personnel managers.

We have also developed three companion computer programs —BBAC, RISK, and ID—which may be used in conjunction with the ideas presented in this book. These programs are described in the text. For more information and for information on how to order these programs, see "A Note on the Companion Computer Programs," which follows appendix 2.

Comments regarding the need for clarity or elaboration in any part of this first edition will be received with thanks. We are happy to acknowledge the invaluable assistance of our colleagues at the University of Toronto and the Addiction Research Foundation. We offer special thanks for the advice given by Dr. Yedy Israel and Dr. Hector Orrego. The reader can safely ascribe errors and omissions to the authors alone.

Acknowledgments

T hanks are given to:
The American Medical Association for permission to reproduce the questions in the CAGE questionnaire. This was originally published by J.A. Ewing, "Detecting Alcoholism: The Cage Questionnaire," in the *Journal of the American Medical Association,* 1984, volume 252, pages 1905–1906.

The Williams and Wilkins Company for permission to reproduce questions in the SAAST questionnaire originally published by L.J. Davis, R.D. Hurt, R.M. Morse, and P.C. O'Brien, "Discriminant Analysis of the Self-Administered Alcohol Screening Test," in *Alcoholism: Clinical and Experimental Research,* 1987, volume 11, pages 269–273.

Cook Critical Care Products for permission to simulate their plastic card reproduction of the Glasgow Coma Scale and Dr. Laurence Dworet, Holy Cross Hospital, Mission Hills, California for compiling the information.

1

Basics

Names

The chemical name for alcohol is *ethanol,* although some writers use the older chemical name *ethyl alcohol.* Ethanol is the most widely known member of a large group of chemical compounds called alcohols. It is the only member of the group that is sufficiently "nontoxic" to be used as a principal active ingredient of alcoholic beverages. Another well-known member of the group is *methanol,* which also goes under the names of *methyl alcohol* and *wood alcohol.* Methanol is the compound that, besides intoxication, causes blindness after consumption. *Isopropanol* is the compound used in rubbing alcohol and disinfecting solutions. Methanol or isopropanol can be added to ethanol to make the ethanol unsuitable for consumption. Such mixtures are called *denatured alcohol.* In this book the word *alcohol* means *ethanol.*

Origin

Alcohol can be produced synthetically. However, most of it still comes, as it has since antiquity, from the fermentation of sugar or starch, in the presence of yeast, in fruits, vegetables, and grains.

Characteristics

Pure, undiluted alcohol is a clear, colorless liquid. It is volatile and so exists partly as a gas that has a characteristic odor. In the purest form, alcohol is almost undrinkable because of its burning taste. It is inflammable, so consumption would not only be unpleasant it would be dangerous. The density of alcohol is less than that of water, although they mix readily.

Uses

Examples of the wide use of alcohol include uses as a solvent, as a fuel, and as an antidote to methanol poisoning (see chapter 5). However, most alcohol produced is for alcoholic beverages.

Units of Concentration

Volume Percent

Concentration units provided by manufacturers of alcoholic beverages are usually volume percent, for example, 20 milliliters of alcohol per 100 milliliters of the beverage. Manufacturers usually state this as "20 percent alcohol." The *weight* of alcohol per unit volume is not often stated, although it is useful for calculations (there are exceptions in places like Germany and Chile).

Proof Units

Although frequently printed on the labels of bottles of distilled spirits, proof units are not in general use. The word *proof* refers to *proof of alcohol content*, and several tests have been used. The most famous test was to mix the beverage with gunpowder; if it merely burned after ignition, then this was proof of sufficient alcohol content. If, on the other hand, the mixture was explosive, then the alcohol content would be described as "over proof."

Clearly, this kind of test will only work on beverages that have a high proportion of alcohol. Perhaps to the dismay of government chemists, tests such as this are no longer used. They have long been replaced by instrumental methods.

Different proof units are used in the United Kingdom and the United States. The net effect is that 1 degree proof means 0.57 percent alcohol in the British system and 0.50 percent alcohol in the American system.

Concentration of Alcoholic Beverages

Legally Produced Beverages

The table below lists most alcoholic beverages and the concentration ranges found in industrialized countries. There are many exceptions to the values quoted in the list. For example, it is possible to find liqueurs with alcohol concentrations up to 60 percent, but they are not common.

Concentration of alcoholic beverages	
	% *alcohol*
Low-alcohol beers	1.2–2.5
Low-calorie beers	2.4–4.0
Beers	3.0–5.5
Strong beers	5.6–9.0
Wine "coolers"	4.5–6.5
Wines	8.5–14
Fortified wines (e.g., port)	17–20
"Digestive" bitters	25–40
Liqueurs	15–40
Spirits	39.5–43

Illicitly Produced Beverages

Illicitly produced beverages, called *moonshine*, or *poteen*, or *potheen*, are likely to have different strengths of alcohol from brew to brew. They are often more potent than their officially sanctioned cousins. The authors have analyzed Trinidadian moonshine rum containing 52 percent alcohol. It is, therefore, about one-third more concentrated than the legal beverage. Although this high concentration of alcohol may surprise the consumer, this should not be the only concern. Out of greed, some illicit producers sell early distillate that contains high concentrations of methanol, the consumption of which sometimes leads to blindness.

Conversion of Units

Many calculations, such as the estimation of a person's blood alcohol concentration, require the use of metric units of volume and weight.

Conversion of Fluid Ounces (fl oz) to Milliliters (mL)

The factor used in this calculation depends on whether you want to convert British or U.S. fluid ounces. To convert from British fluid ounces to milliliters, multiply by 28.4. To convert from U.S. fluid ounces to milliliters, multiply by 29.6. (See appendix 1.)

Conversion of British Gills to Milliliters

To convert British gills to milliliters, multiply by 142. (See appendix 1 for other conversion tables.)

Volume of a Drink

The volume of a drink depends upon the nature and the strength of the drink, and these vary with time, setting, and location.

The following tale of three cities illustrates the variation in volumes of drinks served in commercial establishments. In Toronto, the Addiction Research Foundation reports that the most common servings are:

Toronto		
	(British) Fl oz	*mL*
Beer	12	341
Wine	6	171
Fortified wine	2	57
Spirits	1.25	36

There is variation, though, and in the down-market establishments frequented by the authors 1-ounce servings of spirits are not uncommon. In London, servings of weaker beer are often larger but the servings of spirits are less generous.

London		
	(British) Fl oz	*mL*
Beer (1 pint)	20	568
Wine	4.4	125
Fortified wine	1.67	47
Spirits (1/6 gill)	0.83	24

Regional differences abound; in Scotland and Northern Ireland the servings of distilled spirits are more generous than in England and Wales. And away from the tourist areas of the Caribbean they often serve single drinks of spirits in volumes of 2 to 3 ounces.

A survey of large hotels in Buffalo, New York, yielded the following information:

Buffalo		
	(U.S.) Fl oz	*mL*
Beer	12	355
Wine	6	178
Fortified wine	1.5	44
Spirits	1	30

Note that the servings in the three tables above are for commercial establishments. Servings in the home may be more generous.

The Weight of Pure Alcohol in a Drink

Significance

The weight of the pure alcohol involved is the significant number when estimating:

1. an individual's consumption of alcohol from different beverages

2. an individual's blood alcohol concentration from the amount of alcohol consumed

3. the amount of alcohol consumed from the blood alcohol concentration

Calculation

The weight of alcohol (in grams) contained in a drink can be calculated simply. To do the calculation, we need to know the strength (percent alcohol) and volume (in milliliters) of the drink and the density of pure alcohol (0.789). The formula is:

$$\text{Wt of alcohol} = \frac{\% \text{ alcohol}}{100} \times \text{mL of beverage} \times 0.789$$

Example: Using a generous glass of vodka containing 2 British ounces, take three steps to calculate the weight of the alcohol:

1. Examine the bottle to find that it is, say, 40 percent alcohol.

2. Convert from British ounces to milliliters by multiplying the number of ounces, 2, by 28.4 to give 56.8 mL.

3. Calculate:

$$\text{Wt of alcohol} = \frac{40}{100} \times 56.8 \times 0.789 = 17.9 \text{ grams}$$

A Standard Drink

Standard drink is a term that suggests a fixed amount of alcohol served in commercial establishments. The term is in common use but it is a term that has limited meaning. This is because the alcohol content of a drink varies depending on the beverage, the brand, and the jurisdiction.

The most common servings of whiskey in Toronto, London, and Buffalo, New York contain 11.2, 7.5, and 10.0 grams of alcohol, respectively. By way of contrast, a typical bottle of Canadian beer contains 13.6 grams of alcohol. Cocktails often contain more alcohol than other drinks. A popular recipe in Toronto for a strawberry daiquiri calls for 14.2 grams of alcohol. So, comparisons that involve different beverages, different brands, or political boundaries ought to be made with care. Also, it is easy to see how the use of the British unit system, where 1 "unit" equals 8 grams of alcohol, is not without difficulties.

Alcohol: A Hidden Ingredient

Many pharmaceutical preparations, food flavoring agents, cosmetics, mouth washes, gargling solutions, and breath freshening sprays contain alcohol, and it is not always listed as an ingredient.

Pharmaceutical Preparations

As an example of prescription medicines that contain alcohol, the oral, liquid formulation of cyclosporine contains alcohol at a concentration of 15 percent to help the cyclosporine dissolve. Still, transplant patients on this medication are unlikely to take more than a few milliliters a day. The importance of being aware of alcohol in medicines is emphasized by the accidental poisoning of small children and the situation of adults who are on aversive drug therapy for alcoholism.

"Gripe water" is an over-the-counter medicine in some countries. It is given to babies to relieve spasmodic pain in the belly. Until recently, the preparations typically contained about 5 percent alcohol, that is, about the same alcohol concentration as beer. Now concerns about drunk babies are making governments and manufacturers take another look at the permissible alcohol content of gripe water.

Food Flavoring Agents

Some food flavoring agents contain almost 90 percent alcohol but, as commonly used, the amount of alcohol actually ingested is trivial. Many trifles contain alcohol, but even potent recipes are unlikely to cause significant blood alcohol concentrations.

Cosmetics

Some cosmetics such as perfumes contain almost 100 percent alcohol. Again the alcohol content will only be of importance in cases of mistaken ingestion of large quantities, and this will be particularly important in cases involving small children. The conventional application of perfume or after-shave lotion causes no significant absorption of alcohol.

Oral Hygiene Products

Many mouth washes, gargling solutions, and breath freshening sprays contain alcohol, and some of them contain more than 50 percent alcohol. In principle, use of these products can interfere with the breath analysis of alcohol and cause an artificially high reading. In practice, both the manufacturers and operators of breath analysis instruments know the problem well. Allowing an interval of fifteen minutes between the use of these products and the time of the breath test is usually enough to avoid the problem. During this interval any residual alcohol in the mouth disappears.

2
How Does Alcohol Get into the Body and Where Does It Go?

I N THIS CHAPTER we will consider how alcohol gets into the body (absorption) and where it goes (distribution). This is the first chapter concerning the path that alcohol takes in the body, and our emphasis is placed on practical considerations. In the following chapter we will consider how alcohol is changed into other substances (metabolism*), and how it is disposed of (excretion).

When we speak of absorption of alcohol we mean absorption into the blood system. Absorption of alcohol takes place from most surfaces outside or inside the body but the quantities that can be absorbed through the skin and the mouth are generally trivial. Larger quantities can be absorbed from the stomach, and absorption is most rapid from the small intestine. Significant amounts of alcohol can be absorbed through the lungs if the alcohol is in the gaseous form. This only happens in very special circumstances though, for example, when alcohol is used improperly as a cleaning solvent in industrial processes, and merely breathing the air in the local pub will cause no significant absorption.

The major route for alcohol is from the mouth to the stomach, to the small intestine, to the liver, and then into circulating blood.

---

*Strictly speaking the term metabolism includes absorption, distribution, biotransformation, and excretion. Still, it is common to use the words biotransformation and metabolism interchangeably as in this book.

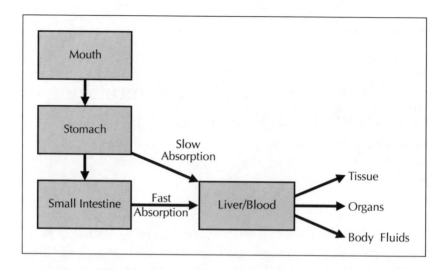

Factors That Influence Absorption

Since absorption occurs most rapidly from the small intestine, any event that alters the movement of alcohol from the stomach to the small intestine will change absorption. There is a large variation between people. There is even large variation in the same person on different occasions with respect to the absorption of alcohol. The most important factor is the rate at which the stomach empties its contents. This is not a very predictable event but we know some factors that are important.

Food

Most people have noticed that the effects of alcohol are more noticeable after drinking on an empty stomach. This is mainly because food delays emptying of the stomach into the small intestine and so slows down the absorption of alcohol. However, the effect does not invariably occur. To avoid criminal proceedings, a person should never rely upon eating to slow down alcohol absorption.

Physical Activity

Another event that causes delay of stomach emptying is strenuous physical activity.

Stomach Removal

The absorption of alcohol can be delayed by events in the stomach. So we would predict that after stomach removal absorption will often be faster. This is what can sometimes happen in practice. There is a surgical procedure called gastrectomy, in which surgeons remove part or even most of the stomach, usually because of cancer or ulcers. Some patients who have had total gastrectomies find that they feel the effects of alcohol sooner than they did before the operation.

Nature of the Beverage

The most important characteristic of an alcoholic beverage with respect to absorption of alcohol is the concentration. Concentrations between 20 and 30 percent (fortified wines), give the fastest absorption. With higher concentrations (undiluted distilled spirits), and with lower concentrations (beer), the rate of absorption is slower. It is slower with high concentration beverages because the opening of the valve between the stomach and the small intestine is handicapped. Alcohol then passes more slowly to the region where absorption is most rapid. Absorption is slower with low concentration beverages simply because it takes longer for the alcohol to diffuse out of the voluminous solution to the walls of the small intestine.

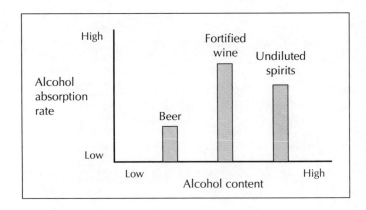

The "Last Gulp" Defense

Here, a person accused of a motor vehicle offense seeks to show that at the time of The Event he had not absorbed the greater part of the alcohol most recently consumed. So, when The Event took place, the blood alcohol concentration was lower than at the time of the alcohol test. (See "A Note on the Companion Computer Programs" following appendix 2.) The computer program BBAC (Blood and Breath Alcohol Concentrations) illustrates the effect of fast and slow absorption.

Distribution of Alcohol into Body Fluids

Fluid means liquids and gases. Breath is the only gas that may contain alcohol that now has significance in legal proceedings.

Body Water

Water is the main component of blood, urine, saliva, breast milk, and so forth, although it is obviously not the only component. Alcohol dissolves easily in water, and, wherever there is water in the body, alcohol can usually be found after the consumption of an alcoholic beverage. The expression *total body water* (TBW) merely refers to the sum of the volumes of the individual components of body water.

The distribution volume of alcohol is affected by the body composition and that, in turn, relates to factors such as age, gender, and weight.

A rapid method of estimating the proportion of total body water in adults is offered in the following rough guide:

Percent body water		
Body type	*Men*	*Women*
Lean	70	60
Average	60	50
Fat	50	40

Example: A man of average build who weighs 75 Kg will have

$$75 \times \frac{60}{100} = 45 \text{ liters of total body water}$$

(To convert from pounds weight to kilograms a multiplication of the number of pounds by 0.454 is required; see appendix 1.)

A more accurate method takes gender and age into account and also uses a more objective evaluation of body type. Height must be in metric units of centimeters (one inch = 2.54 cm). There are two formulas, one for males and one for females.

For males

TBW = 0.336 weight (Kg) + 0.107 height (cm) − 0.0952 age (yrs) + 2.45

For women, age is not an important factor in this empirically derived formula.

For females

TBW = 0.247 weight (Kg) + 0.107 height (cm) − 2.1

Example: A man, weight 75 Kg, height 180 cm, age 60 years.

TBW = (0.336x75) + (0.107x180) − (0.0952x60) + 2.45
 = 25.20 + 19.26 − 5.71 + 2.45
 = 41.2 liters

(These calculations are done for you in the computer program BBAC.)

Estimating the Maximum Concentration
in Body Water

The calculation to estimate the maximum concentration of alcohol in body water from a given dose of alcohol assumes that all the alcohol ingested mixes instantaneously with all the body water. It simply involves dividing the weight of alcohol by the volume of body water.

$$\text{body water concentration} = \frac{\text{grams of alcohol}}{\text{liters of body water}}$$

Example: 20 grams of alcohol in 40 liters of body water.

$$\text{body water concentration} = \frac{20}{40} = 0.5 \text{ grams/liter}$$

Blood

When we speak of blood without qualification we are referring to venous blood, that is, blood in veins. Other kinds of blood include capillary and arterial blood. An important practical point is that while the blood alcohol concentration may be one value, the concentration of alcohol in other liquids will be different. It will depend, among other things, on the water content of the other liquids (discussed below).

Blood Plasma

Strictly speaking, plasma is not a body fluid since it does not exist as such in the body. It comes from blood that has had anti-coagulant added and then been centrifuged (spun at high speed) in a tube to force the red blood cells to the bottom.

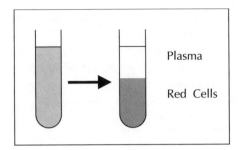

In this figure, in the tube on the right the clear liquid above is plasma. Red blood cells sink to the bottom of the tube after centrifugation. Plasma obtained from healthy persons is a clear, straw-colored liquid. It is possible to obtain venous plasma, capillary plasma, and so forth.

Blood Serum

Like plasma, serum is not a body fluid and it is also a clear, straw-colored liquid. Serum comes from blood in which the red blood cells clotted together before they were removed from the sample.

Other Liquids

Saliva, tears (lachrymal fluid), and urine all consist mainly of water.

Water content of body liquids	
Liquid	*Approximate Percent Water*
Blood	80
Plasma	94
Serum	94
Saliva	99
Tears	99
Urine	99

The greatest variation in water content occurs with blood. The water content varies about 5 percent. Unfortunately, this is the liquid chosen most commonly for the statutory definitions of alcohol concentration used in criminal proceedings. Some uncertainty would be eliminated if instead we used plasma, but this is now unlikely because the use of blood concentration is firmly established.

Erroneous Reporting of "Blood" Alcohol Concentration

Clinical (as opposed to forensic) laboratories commonly do analyses on plasma or serum samples, but may still report the results as "blood" alcohol concentrations. This is sloppy terminology, but it is unlikely to affect medical treatment. It can, however, have legal implications. Two points should be kept in mind for our present interest. The first is that alcohol concentrations in plasma and serum are 10 to 18 percent *higher* than in the corresponding whole blood samples. So a "blood" (really plasma or serum) concentration may appear to be above a statutory limit when the real blood concentration is below it, due to differences in water content of the liquids. The second point is that to obtain plasma, an anticoagulant must be added to the blood sample. Depending on the relative volumes of blood and anticoagulant solution, there may be a significant dilution and, therefore, a *reduction* in the concentration of the alcohol.

Breath

The concentration of alcohol in breath is about two thousand times less than the concentration of alcohol in blood. This is because, at body temperature, alcohol's affinity for water is greater than for air.

Units of Concentration

Unlike alcoholic beverages, it is conventional to express the concentration of alcohol in body fluids as weight per unit volume. There is, though, no general agreement on the units of weight (milligrams, grams, and millimoles) or on the units of volume (mL, 100 mL, and liters). You may come across a variety of units.

We will not explain the scientific term *mole*. It is sufficient to note that to convert from milligrams per liter to millimoles per liter (also known as millimolar) you divide by 46 (the molecular weight of alcohol). Millimolar units are used in some hospitals.

> **The following expressions of alcohol concentration are identical:**
>
> 0.08 grams/100 mL
> 0.08 grams %
> 0.8 grams/liter
> 17.4 millimolar
> 80 mg/100 mL
> 80 mg/dL
> 80 mg %
> 800 mg/liter

We use the style *mg/dL* most frequently in this book for concentrations of alcohol in liquids; *dL* is an abbreviation for deciliter (dl is also an abbreviation for deciliter, but we prefer to follow the international convention).

Breath alcohol concentration units are different because, as noted above, the concentration of alcohol in breath is much lower than in liquids. Units of *microgram*s per 100 mL are in common use. A microgram is one-thousandth of a milligram. The word microgram is often abbreviated as ug, where the letter *u* is the typewriter equivalent of the Greek letter μ. There is more information on the units used for breath alcohol concentration in chapter 7.

Estimating the Maximum Blood Alcohol Concentration (BAC)

The equation for estimating the theoretical maximum blood alcohol concentration (BAC) from a given dose of alcohol is similar to that used for the estimation of alcohol in body water, but we include a factor of 0.80 since blood is about 80 percent water.

$$\text{maximum BAC} = \frac{\text{grams of alcohol}}{\text{liters of body water}} \times 0.80$$

Example: 20 grams of alcohol in a person who has 40 liters of total body water would give a maximum BAC of

$$\frac{20}{40} \times 0.80 = 0.40 \text{ grams/liter}$$

This is the same as 40 mg/dL (multiply by 1,000 to convert grams to milligrams, and divide by 10 to convert liters to deciliters.

This is a maximum because we did the calculation assuming there is instantaneous distribution of alcohol. In reality, alcohol first needs to be absorbed. This takes time, and during the interval there is some metabolism of alcohol. So the theoretical maximum concentration can never be reached.

Breast Milk

The answer to the question, "Can a baby get drunk on breast milk?" is no. Unlike the situation with some drugs, the body does not concentrate alcohol in breast milk. If the mother has a breast milk alcohol concentration of 100 mg/dL and the baby takes 100 mL (that is, 1 dL) of milk then the baby will receive 100 mg of alcohol. If the baby has a total body water of 2 liters then the *maximum* blood concentration that the baby could get from this feeding is 4 mg/dL.

If the same baby took twice as much milk and the mother had twice the concentration of alcohol then the baby could have a *maximum* concentration of 16 mg/dL. Even this concentration is well below the legal limit, and, anyhow, public policy is usually against giving care and control of motor vehicles to neonates. Also, we estimated this concentration on the basis that the milk was taken instantaneously and that there was no time for the baby to metabolize the alcohol. Clearly, this is impossible and the blood alcohol concentrations that a baby would actually encounter even in these extreme examples would be well below the values given above. So, although persistent feeding in this manner may possibly be deleterious to the health of the infant, greater risks would come from other more obvious sources relating to the intoxication of the mother.

Estimating the Minimum Alcohol Ingested

The calculation for estimating the minimum amount of alcohol ingested from a given blood alcohol concentration is just the reverse of estimating the maximum BAC. We use the same formula but we rearrange it for this application.

$$\text{minimum grams of alcohol} = \frac{\text{BAC} \times \text{liters of body water}}{0.80}$$

Here the BAC is in units of grams/liter.

Example: An individual with a BAC of 70 mg/dL and a total body water volume of 40 liters.
   We write the BAC as 0.70 grams/liter. The minimum weight of alcohol consumed is

$$\frac{0.70}{0.80} \times 40 = 35 \text{ grams}$$

This represents three or four commercially dispensed drinks. This is a minimum because the individual would have metabolized some alcohol before the measurement of blood alcohol concentration.

Attempts to Reduce Alcohol Concentration by Drinking Water

Alcohol distributes in all body water and a typical volume of water in a man is 40 liters. (This is the same as the volume of fuel that we commonly put into cars.) So after the consumption of, say, four 250 mL glasses of water, the volume of body water would increase to no more than 41 liters. This is a change in volume of only 2.5 percent, and the same minor effect would be seen on blood alcohol concentration.

Attempts to Reduce Alcohol Concentration by Sweating

Only a very minor effect is possible under normal circumstances, because the volume of water that can be lost in, say, half an hour of sweating cannot compare with the 40 liters of body water. It will not usually be possible to see any effect on alcohol disposition.

Blood Transfusions and Blood Loss

For blood transfusions, the same principle applies as in the above paragraphs. The infusion of 1 liter of blood is a lot since the average man only has about 6 liters. However, this will not make a large change to the volume of total body water. It will not reduce the blood alcohol concentration by a significant amount.

Despite this, blood transfusion can cause a problem in the determination of blood alcohol concentration, if a blood sample is taken downstream from the same arm as that used for the infusion and where both procedures are done simultaneously. Local, temporary dilution effects could cause the blood alcohol concentration to be artificially low.

Blood loss, by itself, has no effect on blood alcohol concentration. It may be helpful to think of a cup of coffee that is partially spilled. The concentration of sugar in the spillage and the remainder is identical.

3

What Happens to Alcohol
in the Body?

M OST OF THE alcohol that a person consumes ends up being
metabolized in the liver. By metabolism, we mean the processes that transform alcohol into other substances. In the main
metabolic system, alcohol is first metabolized into a compound
called acetaldehyde by an enzyme whose name is usually abbreviated to ADH (alcohol dehydrogenase). Acetaldehyde is further
metabolized to acetate by an enzyme called ALDH (aldehyde
dehydrogenase). Acetate can be used by the body for energy.

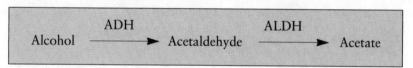

There are secondary metabolic systems for alcohol metabolism
than can be enhanced after chronic drinking. They are responsible, in part, for the increased alcohol metabolism rates seen in
some alcoholics.

Rule of Thumb for "Safe" Alcohol Consumption

If a person consumes alcohol at a rate faster than it can be metabolized, then the blood alcohol concentration will get higher after
each successive drink. The person will eventually become intoxi-

cated. A 70 Kg male can metabolize roughly 10 grams of alcohol every hour, so there is a rule of thumb that says it is safe to consume one drink per hour at a party. If the average drink contains about 10 grams, it is easy to see that the rule of thumb makes some sense. It is also easy to see why people can get into trouble by using this rule of thumb.

Breakdown of the Rule of Thumb

When the rule of thumb breaks down, it usually fails for the following reasons, alone or in combination:

1. Although it is easy to remember "10 grams of alcohol per hour," the average figure for alcohol metabolism is closer to 8.5 grams/hour.
2. The rate of metabolism is roughly proportional to body weight. A woman of 50 Kg body weight may metabolize only 6 grams/hour.
3. There is variation in metabolic rates from person to person of the same weight. It is possible that a 50-Kg woman would metabolize only 5 grams/hour.
4. Many drinks contain more than 10 grams of alcohol.

Example: The drinks served to a woman every hour each contain 15 grams of alcohol. If she metabolizes only 5 grams per hour then there is an accumulation of 10 grams per hour. At the beginning of the fourth hour of the party she would have accumulated 30 grams of alcohol. She would have also just consumed 15 grams for a total of 45 grams on board. This will lead her to have a blood alcohol concentration that is well over the legal limit in all jurisdictions.

Metabolic Tolerance

When we say that a person can drink his friends under the table, we are referring to two aspects of the phenomenon of tolerance.

The repetitious administration of insults to the body often causes the body to increase the efficiency with which it deals with those insults. This effect is called *tolerance.*

For alcohol, the body mounts two main responses: tolerance by the brain, also known as central nervous system (CNS) tolerance (discussed later), and metabolic tolerance. For the moment we are interested in how alcohol metabolism changes with excessive drinking.

The metabolic rate in metabolically tolerant persons can be up to double that of social drinkers. Noticeable metabolic tolerance can be acquired after a couple of weeks of heavy drinking and it can be lost after a couple of weeks of abstinence.

The conclusion that heavy drinking leads to a metabolic tolerance that can be maintained by continued heavy drinking is only true up to a point. Many alcoholics and many alcoholic liver disease patients have normal rates of alcohol metabolism.

Traumatic Injuries

Traumatic injuries are possible after events such as a traffic accident. If there is injury to the liver, for example, or if the blood supply to the liver is disturbed, then assumptions concerning metabolic rate must be questioned if offered in legal proceedings. Appropriate research results will rarely be available because of the impossibility of performing ethical, controlled studies. You will need the help of a good physiologist.

Despite the obvious difficulties, evidence of population average alcohol disposition has been admitted in the trials of severely injured accused persons. There has been at least one unreported case where an accused had suffered a severe liver injury. Since the liver is the most important organ for alcohol metabolism, the fact that the evidence was allowed is startling. Of course, counsel can ask to have irrelevant evidence excluded or can bring evidence in rebuttal. Both routes have well-known difficulties not the least of which is that counsel, trained in one field, must recognize difficulties in another.

Nutritional Factors That Affect Alcohol Metabolism

Low protein intake over a period of as little as a week *reduces* the rate of alcohol metabolism about 15 percent. The effect is reversible if the reduction of protein consumption is not prolonged.

What is a Flusher?

Although it is exceedingly rare in persons of European ancestry, in about 50 percent of Orientals there is a deficiency of the ALDH enzyme that metabolizes acetaldehyde. The deficiency is responsible for high concentrations of acetaldehyde after the ingestion of alcohol. Acetaldehyde has pronounced effects on the body, including shortness of breath, facial warmth (flushing), decrease in blood pressure, and increase in heart rate. These and other effects of acetaldehyde are generally perceived to be unpleasant, so it is easy to understand why this population, called *flushers*, become alcoholics far less frequently than nonflushers. But there are interesting anecdotal reports that some flushers have learned to enjoy the flushing reaction and try to generate it when they drink.

The flushing reaction can be antagonized by antihistamines. So flushers who really want to drink, perhaps for cultural or social reasons, may carry a bottle of over-the-counter hay fever medication.

What Is Endogenous Alcohol?

Endogenous alcohol is the alcohol that occurs naturally in the body without the consumption of an alcoholic beverage. Some medicines, for example, antacids and cimetidine, increase the production of endogenous alcohol in the stomach. These drugs decrease the acidity of alcohol in the stomach and so increase the yeast or bacteria population responsible for the generation of the alcohol.

Concentrations of endogenous alcohol *in gastric juice* seen in postmortem examinations may exceed the legal limit. Still, these concentrations are far below those of alcoholic beverages (5 percent beer is 5,000 mg/dL) and almost all endogenous alcohol is removed on its first pass through the liver. In blood, the concentration of endogenous alcohol does not exceed 1 mg/dL. That is, it does not exceed about 1 percent of the legal limit, and it is therefore only of theoretical importance. Although the chemical entity is the same in both cases, endogenous alcohol is different from alcohol produced artifactually by inappropriate preservation of samples of body liquids.

Concentration Versus Time Profile

The profile seen after a single drink is shown below. The concentrations rise to a peak and then, *in a simple view* of the situation, fall in a *linear* (that is, straight line) fashion until the concentration is very low. Some people describe the shape of the curve from the peak on as a hockey stick.

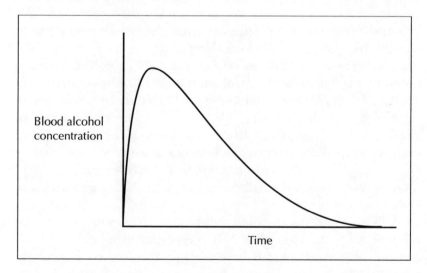

In this simple view, the rate of decline is constant for much of the profile. A rough guide to the rates of decline in different types of drinkers is shown in the table below:

Subjects	Range of rates of decline (mg/dL/hour)
Nondrinkers	8–16
Social drinkers	10–20
Most alcoholics	15–40

Using this simple approach it is possible to *estimate* a concentration at a time in the future. Consider a normal individual who has a concentration of 60 mg/dL on the downslope of the curve. We can estimate that one hour later he or she will have a concentration of 40 to 50 mg/dL. Similarly, it is possible to back-calculate to obtain an *estimate* of the alcohol concentration at an earlier time. However, this practice is prone to many difficulties.

Problems with Back-Calculations

Problem 1

It is important to know whether an individual under consideration was on the upslope or the downslope of the profile at a particular time. The reader will appreciate that for legal proceedings usually only one sample is taken for alcohol analysis. The results of the analysis of one sample cannot show whether the alcohol concentrations were rising or falling. Sometimes, two breath tests may be taken but the usual interval between them, 15 minutes, is often insufficient to allow determination of which way the concentration is moving. This is because the error in the measurements is commonly greater than the small difference in true concentrations seen over a short interval.

Often, the crucial question will be concerned with how long it takes to reach the peak alcohol concentration (see below). This is because once the peak has been reached then the concentrations can only fall.

Problem 2

The linear (straight line) portion of the profile is not really linear, it is a continuous curve. Also, the curve is such that the rate of decline depends on the concentration. So, the higher the concentration, the greater is the "slope." This change in "slope" is illustrated in the computer program BBAC.

When Does the Concentration Reach Its Peak?

The short answer is usually within 15 to 90 minutes after the drink, but times up to 2 hours have been reported. The average time is about 45 minutes. The long answer is that the time of the peak blood alcohol concentration depends upon

1. the rate of *absorption*
2. the rate of *distribution*
3. the rate of *metabolism*
4. the *dose.*

The factors that affect the absorption, distribution, and metabolism of alcohol have been discussed. The way that the amount of alcohol affects the time to get to peak concentration is illustrated in the following figure. Other things being equal, the larger the dose, the longer it takes to get to the peak concentration (and the steeper is the rate of decline). The figure below illustrates the profiles after a single drink and after a quadruple drink.

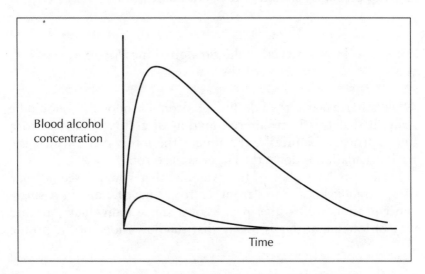

The rate of disappearance of alcohol is mainly determined by enzyme activity in the liver (which may be influenced by previous alcohol use, disease, injury, and other drug use), the distribution of alcohol in the body, liver blood flow (which again may be influenced by disease, injury and other drug use), and blood alcohol concentration.

Despite the complex situation, we would have less concern for one factor, absorption, if the peak alcohol concentration occurred soon after consumption finished. We would then know that the concentration could have only decreased in the interval between the time of The Event and the time of the breath test or the time of a fluid sample. (The Event could be the execution of a will, an assault, or an accident, and so forth.)

It has been said that the peak alcohol concentration occurs within fifteen to twenty minutes after the last drink. This is a misleading statement because it is incomplete. Results have been obtained from many different studies in several different countries from at least 1920 to the present. They show that it can take anywhere from a few minutes to a few hours to reach the peak concentration.

Remember that these studies were done on healthy subjects. If an accused suffers from a disorder that affects alcohol absorption, perhaps because of being injured in a traffic accident, then the effect of the injury should also be considered.

How Curved is the Straight-Line Portion
of the Curve?

When a particular rate of decline of alcohol is quoted, it should be realized that this is an approximation of a curved process to a linear process. Naturally, the longer the interval for which the back-calculation is done, the larger is the error.

Scientists have shown, for example, that you can see a range of apparently linear rates from 12 to 20 mg/dL/hour in a single concentration versus time profile of a single individual. Another way of looking at this is to say that the downslope of the profile after five drinks taken quickly is 50 percent greater than after two drinks taken quickly.

There are ways to describe the curved process by mathematical formulas. They are not in common use, although we use them in the computer program BBAC. The reasons that they are not in use are that

1. You need a computer, a calculator cannot do the job.

2. It is sometimes necessary to know where a subject falls on the concentration versus time profile, although this is impossible in practice unless there is reliable evidence.

3. The processes are sometimes not well described by a smooth curve, or curves.

More on the Dreaded Back-Calculations

It is often the situation that a person has an evidential quality, alcohol analysis done not close to the time of The Event but at some later time. Back-calculations are therefore often used to estimate the blood alcohol concentration at the relevant time.

Under the simplest circumstances, a back-calculation is much like the arithmetical problem of a skier on a mountain. Given that at 3 P.M. the skier was at a particular point (X) on the mountain, where was he at 1 P.M.? In alcohol work, there are often complications equivalent to:

1. The slope of the hill varies continuously and it is generally steeper at the higher elevations.

2. There are different skiers of different abilities and we may not be sure of the type we are dealing with.

3. Each skier takes a slightly different route every time he or she descends.

4. At 1 P.M. the skier may have still been going up the hill.

5. We may not be absolutely certain of the location of point X (transposition errors discussed later).

For an accurate back-calculation, it is essential to know whether the concentrations between the time of The Event and the time of the alcohol test have increased or decreased or have done both. Also, it is essential to know the rates at which the increases and decreases took place. There is no way of objectively determining these events in a particular accused without having reliable information such as the results of an earlier blood sample analysis profile in that individual. These results are inevitably unavailable and anyhow may not be applicable to the situation under consideration.

When Are Back-Calculations Reasonable?

There are several circumstances where the use of back-calculations may be reasonable. The things to look for are:

1. A somewhat *long* interval between the end of consumption and The Event. This ensures that the absorption of alcohol is not a factor in the calculations.

2. A healthy subject. This ensures that there are no complications arising from unusual alcohol disposition.

3. A somewhat *short* interval between The Event and the alcohol test. This ensures that errors arising from the assumption of linearity and errors arising from the use of population mean alcohol elimination rates are small.

Example: A subject consumed alcohol until midnight. At 1 A.M. he started driving home. At 2 A.M. he was stopped by the police. At 3 A.M. he was tested for alcohol and the blood concentration was 120 mg/dL.

The back-calculation here involves adding the average amount that alcohol concentrations decline in one hour. A value of 15 mg/dL is typical. So the back-calculation would show that when stopped by the police the accused's blood alcohol concentration was about 135 mg/dL.

For completion we could use the extreme values for the rates of decline of alcohol concentrations. We know that he is not a nondrinker so the 10 mg/dL/hr low figure for social drinkers is appropriate for the low extreme value. On the other hand he may be an alcoholic who also has extremely rapid metabolism so 40 mg/dL/hr may possibly be appropriate for the high extreme value. This will lead to the conclusion that at the relevant time, the blood concentration was between 130 and 160, with the most likely figure being 135 mg/dL.

On the facts given in this example, it would be difficult to challenge the calculation.

You can use the computer program BBAC to simulate various possibilities.

When are Back-Calculations Unreasonable?

A fundamental question with back-calculations is that, if allowed at all, at what points do the calculations become scientifically unreasonable? There are no scientifically recognized guidelines. The time intervals, the concentrations, and other individual circumstances all have to be considered.

What the Courts Say

A 1987 decision of the Queen's Bench Divisional Court in the United Kingdom in dismissing an appeal from a Magistrates' Court is one that has given some people cause for concern. It was held that the prosecution was entitled to back-calculate from a measured concentration that was well below the legal limit. Although both judges upheld the principle of back-calculation, one of them described the right as mischievous. Press reports at the time indicated that this decision has received little support from the British Medical Association, the Magistrates' Association, and the Association of Police Surgeons.

The Future of Back-Calculations

In the end, scientific truth wins but, as Galileo found out, the process is not rapid. Eventually, it seems likely that in prosecutions, back-calculations will either be subject to very stringent guidelines for their application or they will simply be banned. In the latter case, the alcohol concentration at the time of the test could be made the relevant figure for both prosecutions and penalties. It would then be in the best interests of the prosecuting authorities to ensure a speedy alcohol test. The elimination of costs involved in proving the validity of back-calculations also seems desirable. In civil proceedings and where intoxication is claimed as a partial defense perhaps more leniency could be shown.

Excretion of Alcohol

There is not much that needs to be said about this area. After alcohol consumption, the largest proportion, usually more than 95 percent, is metabolized to other substances. The remainder gets excreted from the body without being altered. Alcohol can be lost from the body as a liquid such as urine, sweat, saliva, breast milk, and tears. It can also be excreted in a gas such as breath. Analysis of alcohol in these fluids allows the noninvasive determination of alcohol concentration. The word *noninvasive* in this context means noninvasive with respect to the body, so that procedures such as taking a blood sample are not required.

Variation in the rate of excretion affects the rate at which alcohol disappears from the body. But since the body loses only about 5 percent of alcohol through excretion, variation in the rate of excretion can only account for an exceedingly small portion of the variation in disappearance rates.

4

Toxic Effects of Alcohol

T O SOME PEOPLE the word *toxic* means a spectacularly dramatic effect on the body such as lethal poisoning. *Toxicity* includes events such as this, but the term also refers to lesser unwanted consequences. Of course, this has still not defined the word. The problem is that the word means different things to different people. Toxicity can mean damage to body tissues. Or it can mean interference with normal biochemical events, interference with normal organ function, or production of disease.

The wide spectrum of toxic effects caused by the inappropriate consumption of alcohol may be conveniently divided into two groups. There are short-term and long-term effects. In both cases, the extent of toxicity depends on the amount of alcohol consumed being too great *for that individual*.

Short Term Toxicity

The figure on the following page conveys messages that are only valid *on average*. At a party, two drinks usually do little harm but after four drinks, especially if taken close together, there may be intoxication. There is also a risk of exceeding the legal limit for driving and other activities. Similarly, taking two drinks a day, every day, won't usually lead to damage to the body in the long term, but with four drinks a day taken in succession there is an increased risk. It must be emphasized that these conclusions are only sound on average. It would be most regrettable if there is a suggestion, for example, that a pregnant woman can safely

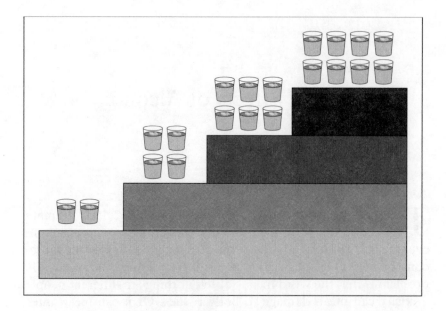

consume *any* quantity of alcohol. Also, some people are susceptible to toxicity caused by very small amounts of alcohol.

The short-term effects of alcohol depend upon the blood concentration. As the concentration increases, the spectrum of effects widens and the intensity of the effects increases.

It is easiest to think of alcohol as a depressant. At lower concentrations, alcohol depresses the functions of the brain that are responsible for inhibitions and control. This results in a reduction of inhibitions and greater activity. Thus it may appear that alcohol is a stimulant but it is not, at least not primarily. At higher concentrations, the depressant effects of alcohol become more obvious.

The following table shows the likely effects in persons not habituated to the drug. It is helpful to remember that there is a very wide variation in the response found in different persons.

There are different grades of coma. Many hospitals use the Glasgow Coma Scale for the ratings; the elements of the scale are listed in appendix 2.

Death from simple respiratory depression is a rare event. Usually the subject would fall into a coma and be unable to continue alcohol consumption long before he or she could drink

Concentration and effect in normal people		
Concentration		*Effect*
Blood (mg/dL)	*Breath (μg/dL)*	
50	22	Mild intoxication. Feeling of warmth, impairment of judgment, decreased inhibitions.
100	43	Frank intoxication in most people. Increased impairment of judgment, inhibitions, attention, and control. Some impairment of muscular performance.
150	65	Frank intoxication in all normals. Staggering gait and other muscular incoordination, slurred speech, double vision, memory and comprehension loss.
250	109	Profound intoxication/stupor. Reduced response to stimuli, inability to stand, vomiting, incontinence, sleepiness.
350	152	Coma. Unconsciousness, little response to stimuli, incontinence, low body temperature, poor respiration.
500	217	Death likely.

enough to cause death. If death occurs, it is more common to see it following another event. This could be a medical complication or trauma.

Alcohol and Trauma

American reports show that there are significant blood alcohol concentrations in approximately

- 50 percent of traffic fatalities
- 33 percent of nonfatal motor vehicle injuries
- 60 percent of fires and burns
- 50 percent of hypothermia and frostbite cases
- 20 percent of completed suicides
- 40 percent of serious falls

These results suggest that physicians should assume alcohol involvement in all trauma cases unless the results of a blood test show otherwise. This is because the common signs of intoxication (slurred speech, bloodshot eyes, and decreased coordination) may be absent and are sometimes unreliable indicators. Still, only half the emergency facilities test for alcohol as a matter of routine.

Tortious Liability of Physicians after Treatment of Trauma

Liability may be incurred by the physician if the patient *subsequently* becomes involved in an accident. This will be particularly true if there was an alcohol analysis at the time of treatment, the concentration was high, and yet the physician offered no advice to the patient concerning, for example, his or her ability to drive.

To avoid or reduce liability some writers have suggested that, besides the oral advice, the patient should be given written instructions. This note should document the blood alcohol concentration and when the concentration should be low enough to allow safe driving. Other observers have suggested that reasonable force should be used to prevent a patient from driving in an intoxicated condition or that reasonable means should be used to immobilize the vehicle.

Alcohol and Sex

The reader may wonder why this paragraph is in the section on alcohol toxicity. The consumption of alcohol has long been practiced in the preliminaries of sexual activity, but there is the phenomenon of "too much of a good thing." Other authors have quoted the bard and we do too. Shakespeare's character the porter said it best in *Macbeth*, ". . . . Lechery, sir, it provokes, and unprovokes; it provokes the desire, but it takes away the performance. . . ." As in many enterprises, nature rewards moderation.

The consequences of not practicing moderation can be grave. The long-term, heavy consumption of alcohol can lead to gender neutralization in women and feminization in men. So it is hard to reconcile the machismo images presented in alcoholic beverage advertisements with the knowledge that persistent heavy drinking can lead to wasting of the testicles.

Gout

Gout is a metabolic disease marked by painful inflammation of the joints. When the body metabolizes large quantities of alcohol, there is interference with the excretion of a naturally occurring compound called uric acid. This compound is then deposited in and around the joints. The process can result in an attack of gout.

Long-term Toxicity

Chronic heavy drinking results in a spectrum of disorders that lead to a variety of clinical signs and symptoms. Some of the signs and symptoms are useful in detecting alcohol abuse and dependence. (A sign is an observable physical phenomenon so frequently associated with a condition that it shows the presence of the condition. A symptom is a manifestation of a condition of which the patient is usually aware.) The following is a survey of some disorders that are important for the purposes of the book, both well known or interesting.

The Brain and the Rest of the Nervous System

There is a wide range of disorders under this heading, including degeneration of the brain. Some of the disorders are detailed below.

Withdrawal from Alcohol. Much of the discussion in this chapter relates to the toxic effects caused by the presence of alcohol, but for some people the absence of alcohol is no joy.

Persistent heavy drinking produces physical dependence on alcohol, and withdrawal can cause serious effects that require medical treatment. Withdrawal reactions most commonly start to occur when the blood alcohol concentration approaches zero. But in a heavily dependent person, a mere decline in blood alcohol concentrations is sufficient to start the reactions.

Depending on the drinking history, a multistage syndrome is possible. Some authors describe a three-stage syndrome while others prefer to characterize a two-stage syndrome (below). It matters little. The essential points are that the reactions are always unpleasant, and they can be life-threatening.

Stage One. This typically occurs in alcoholics after a weekend drinking binge. The drinker may suffer the symptoms of tremor, weakness, cold sweaty skin, nausea, vomiting, and marked thirst. The severity of these symptoms depends on the extent of the dependency on alcohol. Seizures may occur within a day of stopping drinking.

Stage Two. If the dependency on alcohol is great, then a couple of days later the drinker may go into the second stage of alcohol withdrawal. This stage can be terrifying for both the person going through withdrawal and for the uninitiated who try to help. While a subject in stage one may or may not require medical intervention, for a subject in the life-threatening stage two it is essential. This stage of withdrawal includes delirium tremens (DTs, in which intense hallucinations occur), fever, convulsions, and a very rapid heart rate.

Drugs Given in Treatment of Withdrawal. The usual need is to reduce the hyperactivity and stop convulsions, so physicians commonly prescribe tranquilizers and anticonvulsants. But alcoholics who have a history of bad withdrawal reactions may have accumulated a stock of medicines for self-treatment. If nothing else is available then there is always alcohol itself—"a hair of the dog that bit me." Very few authorities recommend alcohol for the treatment of alcohol withdrawal, however.

And Now the Bad News . . . Although a person who has gone through the two withdrawal stages has lost physical dependence on alcohol, he has not lost psychological dependence. Without treatment for alcoholism he probably will continue to drink, and the cycle may be repeated. And just because a person lacks a severe reaction when stopping alcohol consumption it does not mean that he is without serious problems. Severe withdrawal reactions come from a history of high blood alcohol concentrations and often there will be a history of drunkenness. On the other hand, alcoholic liver disease relates to total alcohol consumption that may be at a constant "low" level. Indeed, many French alcoholic liver disease patients have never been severely intoxicated.

Alcohol, Nutrition, and the Nervous Systems. Some people (not scientists, well, not many) use the expression *empty calories* in discussions concerning alcohol. Oxidation of alcohol itself gives 7 calories per gram. Alcoholic beverages, which contain substances other than alcohol, contain up to 500 calories per liter. Yet these beverages have few, if any, of the essential vitamins, minerals, and proteins. Distilled spirits contain almost no calories other than those from alcohol.

If more than half the daily dietary intake is alcohol, as it is in some alcoholics, serious nutritional deficiency effects are likely to occur. These include degeneration of the brain (Wernicke's syndrome) and degeneration of the nerves in the arms and legs (peripheral nutritis).

Toxic Effects May Cause Mental Incapacity. The incapacity may be temporary (see 1 and 2, below) or of a more lasting nature (see 3 and 4, below). Incapacity may arise from

1. Intoxication, while the blood alcohol concentration remains high for the individual concerned. Of course, because of tolerance to the effects of the drug, higher concentrations of alcohol than would be required in normal persons are generally required to produce incapacity in alcoholics. Also note that the extent of the incapacity varies with the alcohol concentration. It would simplify things immensely if scientists could say that you cannot drive properly at a blood alcohol concentration of 100 mg/dL,

you cannot execute a will properly at 200 mg/dL, and you cannot formulate malice aforethought at 300 mg/dL. Yet because of different degrees of tolerance to the effects of alcohol (see chapter 11) no such statements can be made. Also, some psychiatrists believe that no amount of alcohol can negative criminal intent. Still, the usual approach by experts is to examine the observed effects of alcohol in the person. Then they check to see if this is consistent with the measured or estimated blood alcohol concentrations. Lastly they see if the observed effects are consistent with the act or omission or required mental state.

2. Alcohol withdrawal, including a severe hangover

3. Brain damage caused by

   A. direct and indirect effects of alcohol on the brain

   B. a diseased liver's inability to metabolize compounds in the body that are toxic to the brain

   C. exceedingly poor nutrition

4. Mental illness subsequent to alcoholism

Liver

Excessive alcohol consumption is a common cause of liver disease. Alcoholic liver disease includes enlarged liver (hepatomegaly), fatty liver, inflammation of the liver (hepatitis), and scarring of the liver (cirrhosis). There are grades of these elements depending on the severity of the disease. Each element may be present alone or in combination with others. The consequences of alcoholic liver disease depend upon the severity.

The liver is the main organ involved in both the synthesis of compounds that are essential for proper functioning of the body and the removal of toxic substances. So alcoholic liver disease can cause a variety of clinical problems. It can be directly responsible for damage to the heart and the brain, although other alcohol-related mechanisms can be responsible for these disorders.

The Immune System and Cancer

Acetaldehyde, the first metabolite of alcohol, is very reactive. In particular, it forms complexes with proteins. The body recognizes these altered proteins as "foreign" and mounts an immune response. In a small minority of people this response can resemble an attack of hay fever, thus rendering them "allergic" to alcohol.

Alcoholics suffer more from infectious diseases but these are often associated with poor nutrition or poor hygiene or heavy smoking.

Alcoholics suffer more cancers than social drinkers, although it is not always the case that alcohol alone increases the risk of a particular type of cancer. The situation is complex because many heavy drinkers are also heavy smokers, but a few conclusions can be drawn:

1. The combination of heavy drinking and heavy smoking increases the risk to be above that of either activity alone.

2. Alcoholics who are smokers may develop cancers in parts of the body where they are generally not found in smokers who do not drink heavily.

3. With some types of cancer, heavy alcohol consumption is an *independent* risk factor.

Damage to the Fetus

Alcohol-related damage to the developing fetus results in birth defects. The term commonly used is the *fetal alcohol syndrome*, which is often abbreviated as *FAS*. At birth, the baby has a low weight, a small head and characteristic facial features. Infants affected in this way fail to thrive, and there is mental retardation.

There is now recognition that there is often alcohol-related damage that falls short of full-blown FAS. To cover the variety of congenital disorders associated with alcohol use by the mother the term *fetal alcohol effects* (FAE) is used.

Studies up to 1990 suggest that only children of alcoholic mothers can suffer FAS. This is because only alcoholics can tolerate the high concentrations of alcohol required to produce the syndrome. The situation regarding FAE is unclear, and so no safe limit for alcohol ingestion can be given for pregnant women.

There has been speculation that physical and mental abnormalities in neonates can arise from the defects seen in the sperm of some male alcoholics. One study found an association between the father's drinking and low infant birthweight. We need more studies in this area, but it may be that it is not only the alcohol consumption of the mother that is responsible for alcohol-related congenital disorders.

Other Disorders

The variety of problems that often occur after chronic hazardous drinking includes disorders of the heart, bones, pancreas, red blood cells, and stomach. Some of these disorders can be serious; congestive heart failure in alcohol abusers under the age of fifty and fatal stomach bleeds are not uncommon.

Reversibility of Toxic Effects

A Swiss pharmaceutical company has an experimental agent that reverses some short-term effects of alcohol. Unfortunately, not all the effects can be reversed. For instance, the intake of massive amounts of alcohol would still result in death from respiratory depression.

Some long-term toxic effects of alcohol are reversible. Cessation of drinking and treatment can help in the recovery of damaged organs. Scientists at the Addiction Research Foundation in Toronto have shown that even damaged brain cells can recover to some extent. Other scientists at the same institution have developed a drug therapy that is effective in the treatment of alcoholic liver disease. The damage that may be hardest to treat is damage to the fetus, and most authorities presently think that all of this damage is permanent.

5
Effect of Alcohol on Other Substances and Vice Versa

Effect of Alcohol on Other Substances

Alcohol can have effects on other drugs in a variety of ways. In addition, the effects of a single episode of drinking and persistent heavy drinking may be different. First, we consider the possible effects after a single episode of drinking when there is still alcohol in the body.

Absorption

Drug absorption rate can be *increased* by the enhanced solubility of the drug caused by alcohol in gastric contents. But the rate can be *decreased* by high concentrations of alcoholic beverages, which cause impairment of the operation of the valve between the stomach and the small intestine.

Metabolism

Where alcohol has effects on other substances, the most important is interference with their metabolism. This increases the concentrations of the drugs in the body and prolongs the time they remain there. This effect on metabolism can be reciprocal, that is, there can be interference with the metabolism of alcohol (see below). In many situations these are undesirable events. Sometimes the effect of combining alcohol and another drug is modest.

However, the combination of alcohol with drugs that have a narrow margin of safe use can produce dramatic effects. A mixture of alcohol and high doses of barbiturates can be lethal. Indeed, this has been described as the preferred method of suicide for psychiatrists.

What Is a Mickey Finn?

A Mickey Finn is a combination of alcohol and the sleep-inducing drug chloral hydrate. Since the same enzyme system metabolizes both compounds, they can inhibit the metabolism of each other and cause enhanced effects. According to Hollywood lore, the combination causes the victim to pass out very soon after consuming it. The effects of the interaction are not usually that dramatic, though. Also, since chloral hydrate is only available by prescription, the attempted use of the Mickey Finn is surely very rare.

Treatment of Methanol Poisoning

This is an example of the beneficial effect of the interference by alcohol with the metabolism of other compounds. It is a metabolite of methanol that is responsible for causing blindness and not methanol itself. But methanol and alcohol share the same metabolism system in the liver. If this system can be kept occupied with administered alcohol, there will be less chance for the toxic metabolite of methanol to be produced. Meanwhile, methanol will be excreted slowly from the body in the unchanged form. It should be noted that administration of alcohol is not the sole element of the medical treatment of methanol poisoning.

Effect of Persistent Heavy Drinking

In the chronic drinker there is often induction of enzyme systems that metabolize other drugs. These drugs are then cleared out of the body at a faster rate. So increased doses of anticonvulsants, for example, might be necessary in heavy drinkers. Still, while there is alcohol in the body the metabolism of the other drugs may be slowed. This kind of effect, that is, the induction, is also seen in heavy smokers, and since very heavy drinkers are often heavy smokers this compounds the problems of therapeutics.

Effect of Other Substances on Alcohol

It is possible that many drugs have a minor effect on the disposition of alcohol and a few have a major effect. The best known examples are below.

Barbiturates and Phenytoin

Barbiturates were once commonly used as sedatives and hypnotics, but today they have been largely replaced by safer drugs. Phenytoin is an antiepileptic drug. The persistent consumption of these drugs will cause an increase in the rate of alcohol metabolism. Other things being equal, this effect will decrease the blood alcohol concentration at a rate faster than is normal for a given person. After three days off the drugs the metabolic rate of alcohol returns to normal.

Disulfiram (Antabuse) and Calcium Carbimide (Temposil)

Disulfiram (Antabuse) and calcium carbimide (Temposil) are drugs that are sometimes given in the treatment of alcoholism.

What These Drugs Do. The figure below is the same as the first figure in the chapter on alcohol metabolism (chapter 3). It is not alcohol itself that is principally affected by these drugs, instead, there is blockage of the conversion of acetaldehyde, the first metabolite.

The drugs cause increased concentrations of acetaldehyde after the consumption of alcohol. So the therapeutic approach here is to cause adverse effects similar to those encountered by flushers. The effects are intended to encourage the patient to avoid alcohol.

The Reactions. The aversive reactions most commonly felt are flushing, dizziness, pounding heart, throbbing head, and nausea. The potential for these reactions can persist for weeks after the end of drug treatment. Generally, the reactions depend on the amount of alcohol consumed. There is variation, though, in the response from person to person. Thus, even the small quantities of alcohol that are present in some medicines ought to be avoided.

Effectiveness. Perhaps these drugs are effective in the treatment of some alcoholics, but generally the results have been disappointing.

There have been no appropriate, placebo-controlled, clinical studies that show the drugs are effective in causing abstinence from alcohol in most, or even many, patients. Still, such a result might be considered pie in the sky, given the variable nature of alcohol disorders. However, there are lesser but still beneficial effects that are possible.

The best that can be said is that some patients reduce their drinking frequency after relapse while they are taking the drug. Against this must be balanced the problems:

1. There are reports that some patients enjoy the so-called aversive reactions.

2. The adverse effects can sometimes be life-threatening, so the physician must be careful in the selection of patients for this treatment.

3. Patient compliance is a major problem.

4. Disulfiram interacts with the drugs given in the treatment of a variety of disorders. The drugs include those used to treat anxiety, cancer, epilepsy, tuberculosis, and vaginitis. These drug interactions complicate the therapeutics because of the increased risk of unwanted side-effects.

Similar Reactions with Other Drugs. Disulfiram-like reactions are possible if a patient consumes alcohol when taking tolbutamide or chlorpropamide prescribed in the treatment of one form of diabetes, cephalosporin antibiotics, and the antibiotic metronidazole.

The list is not closed. The requirement is that the drug, or its metabolites, be present in sufficient quantities to inhibit the action of ALDH to a significant extent. For this reason, or for the reasons given above, pharmacists now dispense some medicines with a written warning to avoid alcohol consumption.

6

Women and Alcohol

F OR WOMEN, nature has not been generous in the way that the body handles alcohol.

Body Size

Perhaps it is an obvious point, but it is important to remember that women are generally smaller than men. For this reason alone the same drink given to men and women will give higher blood alcohol concentrations in women.

Total Body Water

Even for men and women of the same weight, the volume of total body water is lower in women (chapter 2). The situation may be different if we compare women athletes with sedentary men of the same body weight, but this is hardly an illuminating comparison.

The figure below shows the blood alcohol concentration profiles expected from a typical man (dotted line) and a typical woman (solid line). (This graph is also found as a demonstration in the computer program BBAC.)

In both cases, the amount of alcohol is 20 grams. This is roughly equivalent to a double whiskey. The absorption rates for

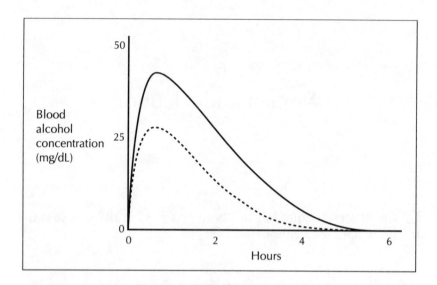

the man and the woman are the same as are the rates of metabolism of alcohol. The ages (35 years) of the two persons are also the same.

There are differences in gender and body size. The man has a height of 180 cm (5 feet 11 inches) and a weight of 70 Kg (154 pounds). The woman has a height of 165 cm (5 feet 5 inches) and a weight of 55 Kg (121 pounds). These differences cause the different profiles. Clearly, the woman has appreciably higher alcohol concentrations over the entire period of interest.

The profiles shown are for one drink given to each person. The position is similar when many drinks are consumed over an evening. When men and women take drinks of the same size, they are effectively taking different doses of alcohol. Using the program BBAC, you can see the consequences of specified drinking patterns. The example given below illustrates profiles that may be expected after our "typical" woman and "typical" man each consume six whiskies, with each drink separated by 45 minutes. (Again, the solid line represents the women, and the dotted line represents the men.)

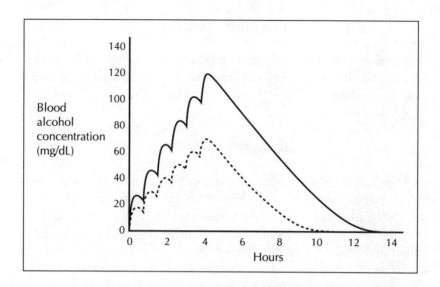

Oral Contraceptives and Alcohol

Oral contraceptives interfere with the metabolism of alcohol; this effect seems to be hormonal. The consumption of oral contraceptives increases the rate of alcohol elimination about one-third. In particular, there is variation of the rate of alcohol elimination during the menstrual cycle of women who are taking oral contraceptives. The rate is greater in the second part of the cycle when the pill is taken. Other things being equal, lower blood alcohol concentrations may be expected during this time. Somewhat higher concentrations may be expected in the first half of the cycle for the same consumption of alcohol.

Menstrual Cycle

Alcohol disposition is similar in women at various points throughout the menstrual cycle provided they are not taking oral contraceptives.

Short-term Toxicity

Short-term toxicity of alcohol is greater in women than in men because the blood alcohol concentrations are higher for the same dose of alcohol.

Long-term Toxicity

Women suffer more extensive damage than men even after considering the proportionately higher effective doses of alcohol. In addition, alcohol-related damages to the fetus, FAS and FAE (chapter 4), are found only in the children of women who have consumed undefinable but inappropriate amounts of alcohol. In addition, alcohol-induced miscarriages can only occur in women. The danger point for miscarriage occurs when maternal alcohol consumption exceeds four to seven drinks a week, but damage to the fetus may occur at a lower level of consumption.

"Behold, thou shalt conceive and bear a son: and now drink no wine or strong drink." This good advice comes from biblical times (Judges 13:7). Unfortunately, until research allows women to know the instant that they become pregnant, they will not be able to take full advantage of it.

Breast Feeding

Breast feeding was discussed in chapter 2.

7

Analysis of Alcohol

Blood Samples

Taking a Blood Sample

A blood sample should be placed in a previously unused, labeled tube and then sealed.

Defense Based on Improper Cleansing. It is a mistake to use an alcohol solution to cleanse the skin area where the puncture is going to be made. It is true that alcohol evaporates very quickly from skin at body temperature. It is also true that studies have shown no contamination of the blood sample when the procedure is done properly. Still, there is a risk that some portion of the alcohol solution will contaminate the sample, and it is proper to challenge the evidence.

Studies on the contamination of blood samples involve taking samples from persons known not to have consumed alcohol recently. When people do studies, it is natural that they would take a little extra care in the procedures. So, these studies are difficult to interpret. On the other hand, it is difficult to have an uncontrolled "field" study. Ethanol that comes from an alcoholic beverage is the same as ethanol that comes from an ethanolic cleansing solution. It is not possible to distinguish the two sources. However, there is another approach.

At our hospital, the Addiction Research Foundation, nurses often use swabs impregnated with another alcohol, isopropanol, as a topical preparation for the removal of blood samples. Sure enough, every now and again, analysts find isopropanol in samples. Usually the circumstances suggest that the only reasonable explanation is contamination of the sample by the cleansing solution.

How Bad Can Things Get? To illustrate the point, let's go back to ethanol. Let us assume that the solution used to cleanse the skin is 100 percent alcohol (more commonly it is 70 percent, but use of this figure only complicates a simple point). A drop of alcohol weighs about 80 mg. So, if one-eightieth of a single drop of the solution gets into 1 mL of blood, the concentration of contaminating alcohol in the sample will be 1 mg/mL. This is the same as 100 mg/dL.

Recommendations. The best procedure for forensic work is not to have any alcohol in the vicinity and to use an iodine solution, for example, to clean the skin. Cleaning with soap and water is an attractive alternative. In some jurisdictions the statutes specify how the skin must be cleaned.

Interference from Other Alcohols. If use is made of another type of alcohol, for example, isopropanol, to cleanse the area, the problem is much smaller. However, the problem only truly disappears if the subsequent analysis is specific for ethanol, that is, ordinary alcohol. If the analytical method measures all types of alcohol without distinction (see below), then there can be very serious problems in the interpretation of the results.

Preservation of Liquid Samples

Artifactual Production of Alcohol in the Sample

One danger to be avoided is that with some urine samples, alcohol can be produced from sugar by microorganisms. This is most likely to happen with diabetic patients' urine samples that are not refrigerated for several days and have not had the appropriate pre-servative added. Most women have bacteria in their urine samples. Diabetics excrete sugar. Bacteria and sugar give alcohol. The preservative that is in common use is sodium fluoride, but it is ineffective against the chief culprit of these microorganisms. So refrigeration of the urine sample is important.

With blood samples collected under sterile circumstances, the danger of artifactual alcohol formation is much less. This is especially true for samples stored under reasonable conditions. Thus, there is no increase in the original alcohol concentration in untreated samples stored for two weeks at temperatures ranging from 0° to 29°C (32° to 84°F).

Artifactual Loss of Alcohol from the Sample

Since sample analysis or reanalysis may be required years later, proper storage is important. Deep freezing after the addition of an antioxidant (which prevents alcohol disappearance) and the use of a good seal seem the best methods.

Analysis of Alcohol in Liquids

There are two basic methods in common use to analyze alcohol in liquids—gas chromatography and a biochemical method that uses an enzyme. There are also other methods, but few authorities recommend them.

The essentials of the chromatographic method are that alcohol is heated to a gas in an instrument and then separated from the other components of the sample by chemical and physical means before measurement. In the second method, scientists take advantage of the fact that enzymes are often smarter than both chemists and physicists in recognizing alcohol. The enzyme used is ADH (discussed in chapter 3) or alcohol oxidase. In this method there is no separation of the components of the mixture. After the enzyme is added, it sets to work on the alcohol, and the progression of the reaction is monitored by an instrument.

The best method of analysis of alcohol in liquids is by head-space gas chromatography. In this method, the air above the sample is first "sniffed" by the instrument. In this procedure, the nonvolatile components of the liquid sample do not have to be separated from alcohol but the remaining volatile components must still be separated. Other chromatographic methods are available, but, in terms of reliability of results proved over many years, this method is best.

An instrument that does the analysis automatically after the analyst dispenses the liquid sample is available commercially from an American company. Still, the instrument costs about $30,000 and is the size of a couple of large suitcases, so it is not suitable for all facilities. If this method has been used by competent and experienced hands, then there is often little point in a detailed examination of the procedures and results. This doesn't mean that the work is unimpeachable. It does mean that you need expert advice on how to do it. The errors involved in other methods of analysis, such as biochemical methods, may sometimes be larger (see below, under "Specificity").

Analysis of Alcohol in Breath

Breath, too, can be analyzed using chromatographic methods. Most of the instruments that are in use today, though, detect alcohol using one of the following methods: thermal conductivity, colorimetric, fuel cell, and infrared absorption. Both the scientific preference of the authors and instrument cost increase in the order given above.

Local statutes define the kind of instrument that may be used to produce evidence for particular purposes. None of the instruments is infallible. This explains why some manufacturers combine two detection methods in a single instrument and use the superior chromatographic methods.

Preservation of the Breath Sample

It is possible to preserve breath samples for later analysis. This is useful if no instrument is available when it is needed for breath testing or if the subject wishes to have the results of the breath test confirmed by an independent laboratory. The statutes of a few jurisdictions encourage this. Several devices are available to keep the sample.

Errors in Instrumental Analysis Alone

There are three things to look for when evaluating errors in instrumental analysis: precision, accuracy, and specificity.

Precision and Accuracy

Precision and *accuracy* are not always understood by those called upon to give evidence. Such persons sometimes get tied in knots when trying to explain the analysis in these terms.

Precision means the variability of the results. *Accuracy* is a measure of how close the determined value is to the true value. So it is possible to have, for example, a very precise analysis that gives a hopelessly inaccurate result.

To appreciate the distinction, imagine a test of two rifles fired by a perfect machine at a target with ten perfect rounds of ammunition in each gun:

The target from rifle one has bullet holes that are (1) close together and (2) close to the center of the target. This means that the gun is (1) precise and (2) accurate.

The target from rifle two has bullet holes that are (1) close together but (2) very far from the center of the target. This means that the gun is (1) precise but (2) inaccurate. We leave other combinations to the imagination of the reader.

Typically, good instrumental methods for the analysis of alcohol have a precision, as measured by the coefficient of variation (CV), of 2 percent. To a statistician, this means that practically every measurement (99 out of every 100) will be good to within 6 percent (3 multiplied by the CV) of the mean value. An accuracy of 2 percent would be satisfactory.

Those readers who have access to a scientific calculator may wish to play with the following numbers: 98, 101, 97, 99, 99,

101, 97, 96, 97, 95. These would be typical results obtained on repeated analysis of a sample where the true value is 100. The first thing that we notice is that the analysis never gave the exact true value although we tried it ten times. It is still a good analysis though. The average of the values is 98.0 and since the true value is 100 then the accuracy is 98.0 percent. The standard deviation is 2.0 (from the calculator) and this yields a coefficient of variation of (2.0/98.0) × 100 = 2.04 percent.

Specificity

Specificity in this context relates to whether the compound analyzed is, in fact, ethanol. Chromatographic methods have very high specificity for ethanol but with biochemical methods the specificity is lower. Other types of alcohol, for example, can give positive reactions. Yet biochemical methods still have pretty high specificity. For example, ADH derived from yeast will not give a false positive reaction with methanol. Biochemical methods are in common use in the forensic science laboratories of the Nordic countries, West Germany, and The Netherlands. Usually the results of these biochemical methods will be accepted in court. Having said all this, we now say that not all biochemical methods are equal.

Differences in Biochemical Methods

There are many biochemical kits on the market and not all are officially approved for forensic use. Medical treatment rarely requires knowing more than whether the alcohol concentration is high, medium, or low. So it is possible that a hospital may use a test kit that is fine for clinical purposes but unsatisfactory for some forensic purposes. It may even be a policy at the hospital to use unapproved kits (and to ignore good continuity of evidence practices) to try to avoid staff involvement in legal proceedings.

The opposite of high specificity is, of course, low specificity, but you can earn scientific brownie points by using the term *high cross-reactivity* instead. If there is any doubt about the method of analysis, then a question concerning the extent of cross-reactivity is appropriate. All biochemical methods of ethanol analysis incidently measure compounds other than ethanol. The issue is one of extent, not fact. You can safely treat testimony that implies that the method measures only ethanol with all the contempt that it deserves. The real questions are what compounds does the method measure inadvertently and to what extent do they interfere in the analysis.

Samples Obtained after Death

It is possible to obtain objective evidence on whether the alcohol concentrations were increasing or decreasing at the relevant time, that is, just before death. This is not an academic exercise. One practical reason for having this information is that the effects of alcohol are more pronounced when the concentrations are increasing than when they are decreasing. The effect is called *acute tolerance.*

In cases involving a fatality, it is usual to have two or more body liquids analyzed. From the ratio of alcohol concentrations in the two fluids it is sometimes possible to tell whether the blood alcohol concentrations were increasing or decreasing. Blood and urine are the most commonly analyzed autopsy liquids, and later in this chapter we describe how the results may be used.

Stomach Contents

A point of confusion may arise in the interpretation of the analysis of stomach contents from deceased persons who had been taking certain drugs. This was discussed in chapter 3 under "Endogenous Alcohol".

Use can be made of the concentration of alcohol in stomach contents to try to figure out whether the deceased was in the alcohol absorption phase at death. No strict rules are possible. This is because the nature, strength, and times of consumption of the beverage(s) taken in the hours before death are usually not known with certainty. Some authors have suggested that a stomach liquid concentration of 500 mg/dL or more *suggests* that the deceased was in the absorption phase at the time of death.

Aqueous humor

Aqueous humor is in the eye. Use is sometimes made of it in post-mortem cases because it is in a somewhat isolated compartment. Therefore, it is less likely to be influenced by putrefaction effects.

Other Errors

Errors involved in the back-calculation of alcohol concentrations are discussed in chapter 3. Errors involved in the transposition of the alcohol concentration in one fluid to another are discussed now.

Forensic Transposition of Concentrations

Because of the large number of alcohol-related accidents that result in death and injury to persons and property, legislatures have passed laws to deter and penalize drunken driving. Prosecutions often require objective evidence of alcohol involvement. The simplest way to obtain this is to get a specimen from the person by noninvasive means. Breath and urine are the fluids most often used. There is now little or no debate concerning the public policy objectives; it is the application of the science that is often at issue.

The problems come from the necessity of calculating a *blood* alcohol concentration from a breath or urine alcohol concentration.

Some readers may be fortunate enough to live in a jurisdiction where enlightened legislators have made this calculation unnecessary by using *breath* alcohol concentrations to define the legal limit for driving a motor vehicle. If so, then this section of the book may be ignored in safety. (At least this is true with respect to motor vehicle offenses. If intoxication is a partial defense to the crime of interest or if the issue is in a civil case then the rest of this chapter may be worth reading.) The combination of certainty of the science and certainty of the criminal law that you enjoy is the envy of your colleagues in less blessed jurisdictions.

How do you know if you live in one of these favored jurisdictions? All that is necessary is to find out whether the local statutes define the legal limit for driving a motor vehicle in terms of *breath* alcohol concentration. A typical *breath* alcohol concentration limit will be about 2,300 times lower than a blood alcohol concentration limit. Unfortunately, because of the bewildering array of units used, it is not always easy to tell.

The following table lists some statutory breath alcohol concentration limits. In the last column the various values are in common units for ease of comparison. Please note that in the United States and in other federated countries the situation may vary from jurisdiction to jurisdiction.

Country	Breath alcohol concentration limit	
Austria	0.40 mg/L	40 µg/dL
Britain	35 µg/100 mL	35 µg/dL
France	0.40 mg/L	40 µg/dL
Japan	0.25 mg/L	25 µg/dL
Netherlands	220 µg/L	22 µg/dL
New Zealand	500 µg/L	50 µg/dL
U.S. (most states)	0.1 g/210L	45 µg/dL

As of 1990, the following countries do not have statutory *breath* alcohol concentration limits although they do have limits for *blood*: Australia, Canada, Denmark, Norway, Republic of Ireland, Sweden, Switzerland, and West Germany.

In some jurisdictions there are statutory limits for the concentration of alcohol in *urine*. In Britain the limit is 107 mg/dL. In U.S. jurisdictions the most common limit is 149 mg/dL (usually written as 0.1 g/67 mL).

There will be more on urine later in the chapter, but for the moment we shall concentrate on breath.

Breath Analysis

Breath Analysis Gives Only Breath Alcohol Concentration

Breath analysis devices used by the police forces in the less blessed jurisdictions usually give a readout in units of *blood* alcohol concentration. Since a breath analysis instrument can only measure breath alcohol concentration, a hidden calculation must occur. This calculation is supposed to transpose breath concentration to blood alcohol concentration. To the question, "Is the calculation any good?," the answer must always be, "Yes, sometimes."

This area is very controversial; the arguments have been going on for decades. There is more case law on the subject than on the constitutions of most countries. Also, the volume of scientific and technical writings is far more than that expected for such a narrow area. The reasons for these phenomena include the widespread incidence of drinking and driving cases and the elements of strict liability involved in most statutes that limit defenses.

On one side, you generally have the Crown or the State and related scientific offices. They say that there are only a few problems with breath analysis and transposition of the results and that they don't usually cause significant difficulties. On the other side, you generally have the academic types, who are more commonly associated with the defense, gasping in horror at the necessary assumptions. It will never be possible to find out the extent to which the situation would be reversed if breath analysis were commonly used as evidence to support a partial defense and very rarely as evidence to support a prosecution, but it might be interesting to speculate.

In a sense, to focus on the issues is to miss the point. Any area that causes scientists to make bitter personal attacks and sometimes act like fanatics is probably an area where there is legitimate doubt. We hope that the information below will inform and stimulate the reader without causing a departure from decorum.

Errors in Breath Analysis

The smallest errors in breath analysis are in the instrument itself and the calibration of the instrument. The largest errors come from *inter*individual variability. In this case, interindividual variability means, for example, that if two people have the same breath alcohol concentration they will not necessarily have the same blood concentration. There is also *intra*individual variability, where breath analyses from the same person at essentially the same time give different results. This arises because no two breath samples are identical. The errors that come from biological variability are not really errors at all. They are only errors in the sense that breath alcohol concentration does not always accurately reflect blood alcohol concentration.

It has been well shown that most of the error in a breath analysis measurement comes from biological variability. Consequently, the estimates of instrumental error given by manufacturers of breath analysis instruments are usually among the least important considerations. So while the authorities make commendable effort to define which scientific instruments are acceptable for breath testing, the effort is, in a sense, misdirected. Most of the error usually arises elsewhere.

Wrongful Conviction, Wrongful Acquittal

The most common way for scientific error to be quoted is by the value of the coefficient of variation (CV), which is often expressed as a percentage. First, consider the error in the transposition of breath to blood. Various figures are available, but we shall take a recent estimate of a CV of 9 percent. Now consider a breath measurement transposed to read a concentration of 80 mg/dL in blood (the legal limit in many jurisdictions). This should be interpreted as meaning that there is a 99 percent probability that blood measurement at this concentration will be between 58.4 (80 minus three CVs) and 101.6 mg/dL (80 plus three CVs).

At this stage it may appear to the reader that we have taken an extreme example. It may be thought to be impossible that an accused with a true blood alcohol concentration of, say, 65 at the time of the offense could be wrongfully convicted. Or that an accused with a true blood alcohol concentration of, say, 100 at the time of the offense could be wrongfully acquitted. In fact, the example is not extreme and the real situation is worse.

What Is the Blood:Breath Ratio?

The blood:breath ratio is the concentration of alcohol in blood divided by the concentration of alcohol in breath. It is this ratio that is used to transpose breath alcohol concentration to blood alcohol concentration. A breath alcohol concentration when multiplied by the blood:breath ratio is said to give the blood alcohol concentration.

The ratio is usually assumed to be constant with respect to time and constant between people. A value for this ratio of about 2,300:1 is often quoted. Many breath instruments, though, use a ratio of 2,100:1 to reduce the number of wrongful convictions at the expense of increasing the number of wrongful acquittals. The transposition of breath to blood concentration is subject to several errors.

No Single Value Possible for the Blood:Breath Ratio

The question often arises about the exact value of the blood:breath ratio. It will be apparent from the discussion below that because of interindividual, intraindividual, and time-dependent variations, no single value exists.

Interindividual and Intraindividual Variation of the Blood:Breath Ratio

Reported ratios vary from about 1,000:1 to about 7,000:1. Still, data reported since 1980 now suggest that the variation in the ratio is less and that typically the range is from about 1,100:1 to about 3,500:1. That is, instead of a sevenfold variation, the variation is more like threefold. This is still not comforting. Much of the variation comes from the time dependence of the ratio.

Time Dependence of the Blood:Breath Ratio

You can understand the principle best by considering the situation a few seconds after consumption. At this time there is a very small amount of alcohol in blood in the lungs but none at all in the venous blood (in the arms, for example). Now, the alcohol in the lung blood can get into the breath. So an analysis for breath alcohol would be positive whereas an analysis for alcohol in venous blood would be negative. Another way of expressing this is to say that the blood:breath ratio is 0. Later, there will be an increase.

In the absorption phase of alcohol, breath analysis consistently *overestimates* the venous blood concentration. When absorption becomes somewhat unimportant, then breath analysis *underestimates* the venous blood concentration. The overestimation and underestimation are often worthy of consideration.

What Is a Deep-Lung Air Sample?

The concentration of alcohol in the air of the lungs varies. It is highest near the surface of the lungs (the "deep" area) and lowest at the "top" of the lungs. Many breath analysis instruments are designed to sample only deep-lung air samples. (How deep is deep?) This is done by making the subject blow long and hard before the instrument snatches a sample of the breath for analysis. So, of the air blown into the instrument, it is only the last little bit that is analyzed. If that last bit of air is not deep-lung air then the determined concentration of alcohol will be low. Other things being equal, this will lead to an *underestimation* of the blood alcohol concentration.

Effects of Advanced Age, Heavy Smoking, and Heavy Colds

The most obvious effect is that some elderly persons simply do not have enough "puff" to complete the test as required by some instrument manufacturers. There are similar difficulties with some heavy smokers and persons who have heavy colds.

Another effect is because the blood:breath ratio increases with age. In young adults the average ratio is 2,300:1 but in old folks the average ratio is about 2,900:1. As stated, these are average ratios, but individual values of 4,000:1 are not uncommon in the elderly. Since a ratio of 4,000:1 is about double the ratio built into many instruments for transposition to blood concentration, the error in this transposition can clearly be enormous.

Partial Samples in General

Always, the analysis of a partial breath sample will give a result that is not greater than a complete sample. In other words, the result of a partial test will be more beneficial to a person accused of a motor vehicle offense than the analysis of a complete sample. If the issue is the partial defense of intoxication then the reverse conclusion is valid.

Defense Based on a Partial Sample

Depending on the jurisdiction, there may be a defense to a road traffic offense if a partial sample has been used. The prosecution will say that the concentration was not less than some value. This may be insufficient if a particular concentration is required, or appears to be required, by statute.

Effect of Chronic Obstructive Pulmonary Disease

Breath analysis underestimates the blood alcohol concentration in patients with chronic obstructive pulmonary disease. The average underestimation is about 25 percent.

Defense Based on Regurgitation

Regurgitation of stomach contents may result in portions of the consumed alcoholic beverage reappearing in the mouth. This state may arise from a chronic disorder or it may be of a temporary nature such as that following an accident. If portions of the alcoholic beverage are in the mouth at the time of the breath test then the analysis will overestimate the blood alcohol concentration. The degree of overestimation will depend upon the extent of regurgitation and the concentration of alcohol in the stomach contents. Two breath analyses given, say, fifteen minutes apart, that give essentially the same result tend to negative a defense of *temporary* regurgitation.

The Burden of Proof?

The technique used in a breath analysis measurement is to use a population mean ratio to transpose breath concentration to blood concentration. Some people argue, a little ungenerously, that the onus should then fall on the prosecution. The prosecution should show that this particular ratio is applicable to a specific accused at a specific time under specific conditions. It is not always clear how to do this with certainty. This is the reason for the attractiveness of defining the legal limit in terms of breath concentration instead of transposed blood concentration.

Slight Physiological Preference for Breath Concentration

Breath concentration more accurately reflects arterial blood concentration and, therefore, the concentration of alcohol in the brain. On the other hand, there are huge differences between people to the effects of alcohol. There are also differences in the same person on different occasions. These differences render the preference of academic interest only. So, a limit defined in terms of breath concentration has essentially no more, and no less, physiological validity in terms of the ability to drive than a limit based upon blood concentration.

Transposition Errors Affect Police Policy

In our jurisdiction, Canada, there is no defined limit for breath so a transposition has to be done. The legal limit for blood is 80 mg/dL. The police know that there is sometimes a problem in getting convictions because of "breathalyzer error," much of which is really transposition error. They also have an associated practice of rounding off the value shown on the breath analysis instrument to the next lowest multiple of 10. So the police will often not bother to advocate prosecution in cases where the breath concentration suggests a blood concentration of anything equal to or less than 109 mg/dL. This value is 36 percent greater than that set by Parliament. (How many MPs knew about breathalyzer error when they passed the law?) If we eliminate transposition errors then only instrumental and calibration errors need to be worried about. Successful prosecutions could then start at the equivalent of about 85 mg/dL. Successful prosecutions could start at even lower concentrations if the limit was deemed by statute to include the remaining normal analytical errors of approved instruments.

Urine Analysis

Here we go again. Same song, second verse. The transposition of urine alcohol concentration into blood alcohol concentration can be done, but great care is needed in the interpretation of results. Again, statutory definition circumvents many problems, but several legislatures have not done it.

The Urine:Blood Ratio

Earlier in this chapter we considered the blood:breath ratio, that is, the concentration of alcohol in blood divided by the concentration in breath. Please note that we have now changed the order so that the blood concentration is the *denominator* of the ratio. We know that this switch causes confusion but it isn't our fault; it's tradition.

As explained earlier, an important determinant of alcohol concentration is the amount of water in the liquid. So if blood is about 80 percent water and urine is about 99 percent water the ratio of alcohol in urine and blood should be about 99/80 = 1.24. Now while this statement may be true, it is incomplete.

Variation in the Urine:Blood Ratio

Variation in the ratio is associated with variation in the time of samples after alcohol administration, the use of void samples (below), and the use of samples in which the concentration of alcohol is very low.

The Significance of the Variation. If the urine:blood ratio is too low then the calculated blood alcohol concentration will be too high, and vice versa.

Time. The concentration of alcohol in urine lags behind the concentration of alcohol in blood. So, soon after consumption the ratio is relatively low and long after consumption the ratio is relatively high.

Note that during the absorption phase the use of urine will lead to an *underestimation* of blood concentration. As seen earlier in this chapter, the use of *breath* in the same situation leads to an *overestimation* of the blood concentration.

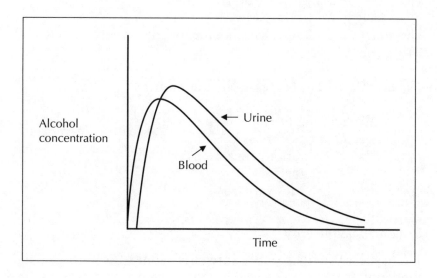

Void and Second Urine Samples. The term *void* in this context means *invalid*, because it is the first urine sample. Naturally, this consideration will not apply where a statute defines the maximum allowable alcohol concentration in *any* urine sample. Void also means that the subject gives this sample to *empty*, or *void*, the bladder 'before he or she gives a second urine sample, sometime later, for alcohol analysis.

For the transposition of urine alcohol concentration into blood alcohol concentration, it is the second sample that is the sample of choice. Analysis of the second sample yields the average urine alcohol concentration from the time of the first urine sample to the time of the second urine sample.

Time and Low Alcohol Concentrations. To understand these problems, imagine the position long after the consumption of alcohol. At this time, alcohol has disappeared from the blood but a little remains in the urine. The ratio of alcohol concentrations in the urine and blood is an infinitely large number. In a case where alcohol has not disappeared completely, the concentration is exceedingly low. So a small analytical error (in absolute terms) can lead to a huge change in the urine:blood ratio.

The Worst Cases. Ratios have been reported that vary from 0.1 to 10 and more.

The Best Cases. The best cases are those where

1. Alcohol is in the elimination phase;
2. Second samples are used; and
3. The concentrations are reasonably high.

In these cases, the ratios vary from 1.1 to 1.5.

Urine Sample Integrity

The issue of urine sample integrity comes up with boring regularity. It matters not whether the issue involves drug use in international sporting events or motor vehicle offenses. There are two elements of importance. The first is that observation of the subject during sampling is necessary. This ensures that the subject does not adulterate (for example, by *dilution*) the sample in any way and that the sample given is *his*. The second element applies to all samples and not just urine: the sample must be secured and preserved appropriately.

Urine Samples in the "Last Gulp" Defense

Here, a person accused of a motor vehicle offense seeks to show that at the time of The Event he had not absorbed the greater part of the alcohol most recently consumed. So, when The Event took place, the blood alcohol concentration was lower than at the time of the alcohol test.

Objective evidence to support or refute the contention may be available if both the void and the second urine samples are analyzed. Much depends, of course, on the wording of the local statutes. A defense on this ground requires that the concentration of alcohol in the second sample be greater than in the void sample.

Similarly, evidence concerning the contention may be available if both blood and urine samples are analyzed. The concentration of alcohol in the blood is higher than in urine during the absorption phase and it is lower after absorption. Naturally, corrections should be made for differences in the water content of the two liquids.

It is as well to remember that these tests may give information on absorption at the time of sampling and not at the time of The Event. Still, on occasion, they can provide useful information.

Recommendations for Reform: Statutory Definition for All Body Fluids

A few points are worth noting about our recommendation to define statutory limits for all body fluids:

1. The key point is that statutory definition of alcohol concentration limits in individual fluids avoids transposition to blood alcohol concentration.

2. Transposition is both uncertain and unnecessary.

3. An obvious alternative would be to use only blood samples for analysis for road traffic offenses. However, the utter impracticality of this approach renders further consideration unnecessary.

4. It may be considered that defining breath and urine limits as well as a blood limit is effectively using statutory provisions instead of "scientific methods" to do the transpositions. This is true. It is also true that there are no reliable scientific methods to do the transpositions.

5. Limits can be defined in terms of the alcohol concentration in urine (some jurisdictions define limits for urine now), serum, plasma, saliva, cerebrospinal fluid, and lachrymal fluid. We also suggest that statutes define *blood* as blood taken from any vessel in the body. This would avoid potential problems caused by differences in alcohol concentration in venous, arterial, and capillary blood and between similar vessels on opposite sides of the body.

   At present, the probability seems low that some of these fluids would be analyzed for alcohol in legal proceedings. Their inclusion is for completeness and to allow for unpredictable advances in research. Data are available to allow statutory definition of limits for all body fluids.

6. It is impossible for some people to give an adequate breath sample because of a medical abnormality or simply because of being elderly. In one report, 10 percent of patients studied in a general medical practice were unable to provide an adequate breath sample. The production of a urine or saliva sample may not be difficult for these people.

7. The donation of a urine or saliva sample avoids the risks, admittedly slight, of bruising and infection that are present

in taking a blood sample. There is also a reduction of risk of infection by the persons who take and otherwise deal with blood samples. In these days of AIDS, this last consideration is significant.

8. Statutory equivalence could simplify a prosecution. Consider a sample of blood taken from an unconscious patient for medical purposes and immediately transformed by a technician into blood plasma. There are two obvious options. A police officer can go through the procedure necessary to obtain and seize another blood sample or he can arrange to seize a portion of the plasma sample. In the latter case it is now necessary to prove by expert testimony how plasma concentration can be transposed into blood concentration.

8
Traffic Accidents

Alcohol and the Risk of a Traffic Accident

Alcohol can effect the skills, judgment, and attitudes required for safe driving. In one sense, the relationship between alcohol and accidents is a very simple one: the more alcohol then the greater the chance of an accident. In accident surveys, scientists confirm this relationship time and time again. Beneath this simple relationship, though, there are complexities.

There is no linear relationship between alcohol concentration and risk. As an extreme example, three hours after the consumption of one beer there is still alcohol in the body. Yet such small concentrations have never been shown to affect the risk of a car accident. At the other end of the extreme scale, when the blood alcohol concentration is exceedingly high, the risk may also be low. This is because the subject may be comatose and incapable of even approaching a car.

Between these two extreme examples the situation is clearer but not simple. There is still no linear relationship. Higher alcohol concentrations in drivers are associated with a *disproportionately* increased risk of an accident. The following graph, derived from the Grand Rapids traffic study, is often shown because it well illustrates this effect.

On average, once the blood alcohol concentration is above 40 mg/dL (about two drinks) then bad things are more likely to happen. This is one reason that some jurisdictions have a legal limit of 50 mg/dL. The effect is not confined to drivers. For example, pedestrians with a blood alcohol concentration over 80

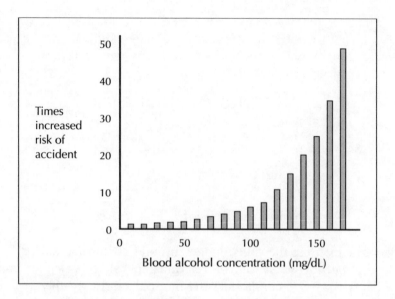

mg/dL are three times more likely to sustain injuries in road traffic accidents. So in a case involving vehicular injury and a pedestrian, it is advantageous to know, or estimate, the blood alcohol concentrations of both the driver and the pedestrian.

There are difficulties in any approach to the legal limit. Age, personality, distance driven per year, level of education, race, nationality, marital status, occupational status, drinking frequency (tolerance), and gender have all been identified as risk factors. Still, public policy would be against consideration of many of these factors when insurance premiums or criminal or civil penalties are contemplated. In any case, when the blood alcohol concentration is high, the other factors are of minor importance.

The RISK Computer Program

The RISK computer program is derived from the results of a major traffic accident study. It allows the user to estimate the risk of a car crash particularly after the consumption of alcohol.

To obtain the program follow the instructions given in the section "A Note on the Companion Computer Programs," which follows appendix 2.

The program can be used by anyone, of course. But we wrote it so that a lay person can use it and understand why he was, or is, at risk. This explains the use of the word *you* in the program instead of *your client* or even *your prisoner*!

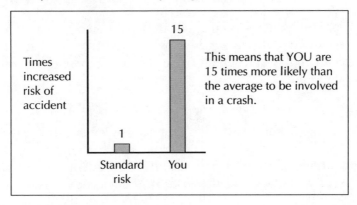

What Information Does the Program Require?

The program asks for

1. information on things that affect the risk of an accident such as age, education, marital status, and current driving experience

2. information on the way alcohol is likely to be handled by the body in question: age, height, weight, and gender

3. information about how the client might consume (or did consume) alcohol at a party or at home, that is, the number of drinks consumed over a stated period

What Does the Program Show?

The program is designed to show that

1. The consumption of alcohol can increase the risk of an accident far more than the variations in risk associated with age, driving experience, and so forth.

2. In young and elderly drivers the consumption of alcohol is especially dangerous.

3. It is possible to avoid excessive risk. There is not too much that can be done simply about age, driving experience, marital status, or education but much can be done about drinking sensibly.

This program assumes simple, linear alcohol metabolism at a rate of 10 mg/dL/hr. This rate is low, as 15 mg/dL/hr is closer to the average for males and females. We thought it best to err on the side of caution.

"The Morning After" and Driving

Clearly, driving while suffering the effects of a hangover increases the risk of a traffic accident. Also, it is not generally recognized that there may be a factor that originates from the cause of the hangover. It is possible that there is a significant blood alcohol concentration even after eight hours of sleep. We describe the computer program for this type of estimation in the next chapter.

The following graph shows the expected blood alcohol profile of an average man who consumed 26 ounces of whiskey between 8 P.M. and midnight. Admittedly, this amount of alcohol is large, but unfortunately consumption at this level does occur sometimes.

The graph illustrates that this person should not drive at 8 A.M. with or without a hangover.

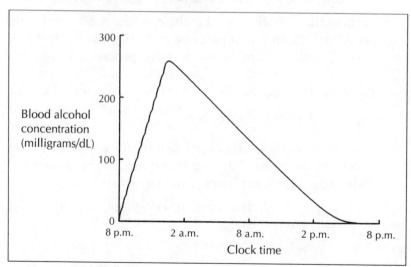

9

Program for Estimating Blood and Breath Alcohol Concentrations (BBAC)

T HE READER is now aware of some of the limitations of calculations in this field. Still, it is interesting to see the estimated consequences of different patterns of drinking and the BBAC program offers a guide.

To obtain this program follow the instructions given on the pages following appendix 2. The program is self-guiding, but for those who are unfamiliar with this type of work we shall run through the most complex part with some simple data.

Using BBAC: An Example

We shall use as our information two drinks, one whiskey and one beer, taken by an average man. If you can work through the program for two drinks, then you should have few problems with more complex information, and you should have no problems at all with the simpler options in the program. On this first run we suggest that you follow our suggested data exactly. In this way, you can check the graph that you get against ours.

The First Screen

This is the title screen. At the top of the screen are the words, "Program BBAC." At the bottom of the screen are the words, "Hit any key to continue." We press the *ENTER* key to get to the . . .

Next Screen

This is the main menu. Since we want to see the result of two drinks we need option 2. We use the number keys at the top of the keyboard and not those on the right-hand side. We type 2 and then press the *ENTER* key.

Next Screen

This screen first asks for the gender. Our subject is a male so we type *1* and press the *ENTER* key.

We would like to give his height in feet and inches, so we type *2* and press the *ENTER* key. Our man has a height of 5 feet 10 inches. We type *5* and press the *ENTER* key. We then type *10* and press *ENTER*

We would like to give the weight of our man in pounds so we type *2* and press the *ENTER* key. For the weight we type *154* and press *ENTER*

For his age, we type *35* and then press *ENTER*

Now we are asked about the metabolic rate of alcohol in our average man. We type *2* and press *ENTER*

We are then asked if the information is correct. Type *y* (it doesn't matter whether you use uppercase or lowercase) if the information is correct and then press *ENTER*

We don't want to get into the Advanced Mode so we type *n* and then press *ENTER*

Next Screen

The computer is asking for information on the first drink. For this drink we are not going to put in our own detailed information. Instead we are just going to use an average drink of whiskey. We type *2* and then press *ENTER*

Next Screen

Here we see that there is no such thing as an average drink of whiskey! The screen is showing common servings in three countries. Since our hypothetical subject is in Canada, we type *1* and then press *ENTER*

Next Screen

Now the computer is asking for the absorption rate. We don't know the answer, but perhaps the drinking was done on an empty stomach and we guess that absorption is fast. So, we type *1* and then press the *ENTER* key. We have now entered all the information on the first drink.

Next Screen

Is there another drink (Y/N)? Yes, there is. We type *y* (it doesn't matter whether you use upper case or lowercase for the letter) and then press the *ENTER* key. There is a note here where we are told that you can put in up to fifty different drinks.

Next Screen

Here we have to put in the time after the start of the previous drink. Perhaps it was an hour and 45 minutes. We type *1* and press the *ENTER* key. Then we type *45* and press *ENTER*

Next Screen

For the second drink, a beer, we are going to put in our own information. We type *1* and then press *ENTER*

Next Screen

You are asked for the alcohol concentration of the drink. If you had the bottle handy it would be a simple task to get this information. Alternatively, you could look it up in the table that you have put into the book in the following pages, which were designed for this purpose. This route is unlikely to be fruitful as you have only just gotten the book. The screen in front of you suggests that the concentration of beer is between 3.0 and 5.5

percent alcohol, but we have to be more precise. We need help. So, as suggested on the screen, we press the key labeled *F2*

Next Screen

There are hundreds of beers on the market and the program cannot contain a listing for every beverage. A few brands are on this screen, but the authors readily admit that this help is meager. Also, you must remember that the same brands of beverage may have different alcohol concentrations in different countries. So, Budweiser beer commonly contains 3.5 percent alcohol in the United States but 5 percent alcohol in Canada. Similarly, whiskey sold for export at Heathrow airport (43 percent alcohol) has a higher alcohol concentration that the "same" product sold domestically (40 percent alcohol). This emphasizes the fact that you must get a list of concentrations of the beverages most popular in your area and then write them in the book.

Let's say that the beer is Molson Canadian, that is 5 percent alcohol. We don't need to type anything because this screen is a help screen. At the bottom of the screen are the words, "Hit any key to continued." We press the *ENTER* key to get to the . . .

Next Screen

Now we are back at the percent alcohol screen. We type *5* and then press *ENTER*

Next Screen

Here you have more than thirty-three options for the volume of the drink. We would like help so we press the key labeled *F2*

Next Screen

This screen says that a bottle of beer in Canada has a volume of 12 British fluid ounces. We don't need to type anything because this screen is a help screen. At the bottom of the screen are the words, "Hit any key to continue." We press the *ENTER* key to get to the . . .

Next Screen

Now we are back at the volume screen with the many options. Option 15 is the option for a volume of 12 British ounces. We type *15* and press *ENTER*

Next Screen

We are now asked about the absorption rate for this drink. We type *2* and then press the *ENTER* key. We have now entered all the information on the second drink.

Next Screen

Is there another drink (Y/N)? We are only going to put in two drinks for this practice session. We type *n* (uppercase or lowercase) and then press the *ENTER* key.

Next Screen

This screen says, "Please wait." If you have a fast computer or a computer with a mathematics coprocessor then this screen will only be visible for a couple of seconds. During this period hundreds of calculations take place. If you have a slow computer you may be stuck here for about half a minute.

Next Screen

On this run, we are only interested in *blood* alcohol concenrations so we type *1* and press *ENTER*

Next Screen

This is the graph.

If you got the same as that shown below then all went well. Congratulations. You will now be able to find your way around the rest of the program on your own.

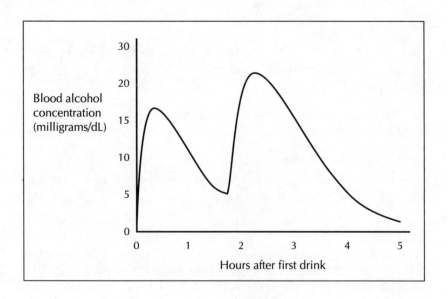

General Remarks

Although you are now a pro, there are a couple of things which are detailed below, to keep in mind when you run the program.

The Time Taken over a Drink

Usually when a person drinks he does so over a decent interval, not all in one gulp. Yet the program is written for gulpers. This will not usually cause a problem and, anyhow, there is a way around it.

Consider the consumption of a 40 mL glass of whiskey over a period of 15 minutes. You can enter this drink as a single 40 mL drink. Alternatively, you can, for example, enter four 10 mL "drinks" taken 5 minutes apart. You can even enter smaller "drinks" taken closer together. You will rapidly discover that entering drinks in this manner is tedious. Fortunately obsessive-compulsive conduct such as this is only necessary in rare circumstances and then usually only for the last drink.

What if the Calculation Is Wildly Different from the Evidence of Drinking?

The two most obvious reasons for discrepancies are a flawed calculation or flawed evidence. A note on the second cause follows.

The Evidence of the Accused. Generally, when an accused starts off by giving a completely accurate account of his drinking it causes surprise to experts. The obvious reasons for an accused's inaccuracy are lapses of memory and his perceptions. Often his perceptions are that less is better for driving-related offenses and that more is better for a partial defense. Experience shows that discussing a reasoned calculation with an accused can do wonders for the memory. Show for example that 1. The accused could not possibly have consumed only four drinks; 2. Six is a more valid number; and 3. Half these drinks were likely "doubles", aids the quality of discussions immeasurably.

The following pages are left so that you can put in the alcohol concentrations of various beverages sold in your area.

BRAND NAMES   **% ALCOHOL**

Beers

_____   _____

_____   _____

_____   _____

_____   _____

_____   _____

_____   _____

_____   _____

_____   _____

_____   _____

_____   _____

_____   _____

_____   _____

_____   _____

_____   _____

_____   _____

_____   _____

_____   _____

_____   _____

_____   _____

BRAND NAMES   **% ALCOHOL**

Wines

_____   _____

_____   _____

_____   _____

_____   _____

_____   _____

_____   _____

_____   _____

_____   _____

_____   _____

_____   _____

_____   _____

_____   _____

_____   _____

_____   _____

_____   _____

_____   _____

_____   _____

_____   _____

_____   _____

BRAND NAMES % **% ALCOHOL**

Spirits

_____ _____
_____ _____
_____ _____
_____ _____
_____ _____
_____ _____
_____ _____
_____ _____
_____ _____
_____ _____
_____ _____
_____ _____
_____ _____
_____ _____
_____ _____
_____ _____
_____ _____
_____ _____
_____ _____

BRAND NAMES   **% ALCOHOL**

Liqueurs

_____   _____

_____   _____

_____   _____

_____   _____

_____   _____

_____   _____

_____   _____

_____   _____

_____   _____

_____   _____

_____   _____

_____   _____

_____   _____

_____   _____

_____   _____

_____   _____

_____   _____

_____   _____

_____   _____

10
Identification of Alcoholics in Legal Proceedings

The Importance of Identifying an Alcoholic

The prevalence of alcoholism in the general population is only a few percent. So, in day-to-day living most people rarely encounter an alcoholic, although much depends on the definition of alcoholism. However, once we move into the realm of legal proceedings, things are different. The prevalence of alcoholism is much greater in defendants and accused persons, since these people often attain their status because of the detrimental effects of the disorder. Half the cases of homicide and up to a third of the cases of child abuse are associated in some way with the use or abuse of alcohol. Yet alcoholism is a condition that sometimes passes unnoticed by all except the individual's family.

There are many reasons why the presence of alcoholism may need to be established. They include the rebuttal of evidence of good character in criminal proceedings and in civil cases when the character of the plaintiff is an issue. Still, alcoholism, without qualification, may be no more evidence of bad character than flat feet. On the other hand, alcoholics, as a group, are involved in violent incidents and suffer from sickness far more frequently than the rest of the population.

In this book, we don't consider nonlegal proceedings, such as "screening" to exclude alcoholics from employment, because of the complex human rights and logical issues involved. The approach that we suggest will work best for evidence given under oath in an adversarial situation or given in confidence during a privileged conference.

"It Takes One to Know One". . .Or Does It?

We apply this old phrase to all kinds of character traits and, no doubt, some people apply it to alcoholism. But if there is an implication that nonalcoholics cannot identify alcoholics then it is untrue. Alcoholics can be identified by nonalcoholics, and identification is possible without the use of either heroic measures or impossibly subtle techniques.

The General Method

Persistent heavy consumption of alcohol usually leaves marks on the body and the mind of an alcoholic and they travel with him always. It is these marks that allow identification. The technique used will be familiar to investigators who have studied the law of fraud. An investigator examining a possible fraud case would be particularly interested in a disposition stated to be made "without fraudulent intent." An investigator interested in alcoholism will be particularly interested in bone fractures and head injuries. It is possible, of course, for an honest disposition to include the above statement. It is also possible for a nonalcoholic to have had bone fractures and head injuries in his adult life. In both cases, though, suspicions should arise that may be confirmed or denied by further investigation.

What Approaches Are Impractical?

Since the reader is unlikely to be a physician, a clinical examination is not possible. This does not matter too much, since the missed diagnosis of alcoholism by physicians is very common.

Next, the results of blood tests for alcoholism are often not available since they may have to be ordered and consented to. The results of a blood (or other) test for alcohol (as opposed to alcoholism) may be available and is a good place to start. Or it would be if we could first define what we are seeking.

What Is an Alcoholic?

At some time, many readers will have grappled with the question, "What is law?" and may therefore have sympathy for the authors in this section of the book. Even when we exclude religious or moral overtones, the definition of alcoholism depends upon time, location, and the bias of the author. Always, though, the term *alcoholic* refers to a person who suffers significant deleterious consequences from his association with alcohol.

As an example of temporal and cultural influences on the perception of hazardous drinking, consider the campaign in France in the 1950s. The officially approved slogan was, "Practice moderation—No more than three liters of wine per day!" Nowadays, research shows that the consumption of far less alcohol can cause problems, and the definitions of what constitutes an alcoholic vary accordingly.

The reader should note that the modern tendency among scientists is to use terms *alcohol abuser* and *alcohol-dependent person* (see below) instead of the term *alcoholic*. Obviously though, the term alcoholic is going to be in use for a long time to come. A list of problems and definitions follows that are useful for characterizing persons. They are useful for understanding both expert testimony and the results of various tests, which are described in the following chapter.

Sociological Problems

Intoxication resulting from the consumption of more than four drinks in succession, three days a week, every week, is often associated with problems for the male drinker. (The consumption figures for women are about 25 percent lower.) Yet some people would call this level of drinking normal, others would call it hazardous or heavy or problematic, and others would call it pre-alcoholic.

Physiological Problems

Physiological problems are based upon the amount of alcohol required to cause organ damage. The long-term, daily consumption of 80 grams (about six drinks) of alcohol undoubtedly increases the risk of organ damage in men. Other investigators have found that 60 grams is the amount for men and that the daily consumption of 40 grams of alcohol causes organ damage in women. Finally, there is a report (from France) that says that 40 grams per day in men is enough to cause increased risk of cirrhosis.

The WHO Definition of Alcoholism

The World Health Organization defines (in part) dependence on drugs as, "A state, psychic and sometimes also physical, resulting from the interaction between a living organism and a drug, characterized by behavioral and other responses that always include a compulsion to take the drug on a continuous or periodic basis to experience its psychic effects, and sometimes to avoid the discomfort of its absence. Tolerance may or may not be present." This definition encompasses the notions that dependence on alcohol includes a wish to continue drinking, withdrawal reactions if drinking stops, and the likely presence of tolerance.

A Psychiatric Definition

The American Psychiatric Association's DSM-III-R (*Diagnostic and Statistical Manual of Mental Disorders Revised*) defines an alcoholic as an individual engaging in the continuous consumption of alcohol despite resulting social, occupational, psychological, or physical problems. This definition also includes recurrent alcohol use in situations when it is hazardous, for example, recurrent episodes of driving while intoxicated.

The NCA Criteria

The National Council on Alcoholism in the United States has published criteria for the diagnosis of alcoholism. Alcoholism can be established, it says, if one or more of the major criteria or if several minor criteria are present.

The problem with this instrument is that it is complex. The NCA report has ninety-one criteria and requires a medical history, physical examination, and laboratory data. Because it is complex, the full instrument is not in widespread use, but some major criteria are useful. For example, a blood alcohol concentration of more than 150 mg/dL without the person showing evidence of intoxication may be sufficient to diagnose alcoholism (see chapter 11).

The Modern Trend

These days, scientists distinguish between alcohol abusers and alcohol-dependent persons according to the following scheme:

	Social/medical problems	*Dependence, impaired control*
Alcohol abuse	+	—
Alcohol dependence	+	+

Alcohol abusers suffer a variety of social and medical problems. They are neither physically nor psychologically dependent on alcohol. "Problem drinker" is another term for a person in this category.

Alcohol-dependent persons have social and/or medical problems and they are also dependent on the drug. They may show marked tolerance to alcohol and withdrawal symptoms after drinking stops. These persons have a reduced ability to control drinking behavior.

The categories are not entirely discrete, and there may be a time factor so a person may shuttle between the two groups during his drinking history.

Distinguishing between persons who merely abuse alcohol and those who are dependent on the drug is important in modern approaches to treatment (discussed in chapter 12). Anyhow, in the minds of the authors, the label *alcoholic* has no moral significance; it is merely a psycho-social-medical description. When scientists use the term *alcoholic*, they usually take it to mean an alcohol-dependent person.

Social drinkers have no social or medical problems related to their consumption of alcohol. They are always in control of how much alcohol they consume and both when and where they consume it. Typically, they consume six or fewer drinks per week and no more than two drinks per occasion.

Finally, it is interesting to note that the average consumption of persons admitted for the first time for treatment of alcohol-related problems at the Addiction Research Foundation is about sixty drinks a week.

Is You Is or Is You Ain't . . . an Alcoholic?

When we say that a person is an alcoholic we should qualify the words by saying how certain we are of the conclusion. Various standards are possible, but we shall start the discussion with the test used in criminal law, that is, beyond reasonable doubt.

The problem is that "beyond reasonable doubt" has limited meaning in a scientific area. Here, studies usually involve groups of people instead of individuals and numerical probabilities instead of definitive statements. Now when an investigator tries to identify an alcoholic, he is embarking, at least in part, on a scientific path. So it is appropriate to understand the scientific limitations of the methods used.

Perhaps it is reasonable to say, in some circumstances, that in science "beyond reasonable doubt" means being right nineteen times out of twenty. This is the test used in most public opinion surveys. Perhaps this test is unreasonable. Surely subscribers to the realist school would insist that the standard of proof varies with the gravity of the criminal charge. Few readers would say that it was sufficient to be right about an important piece of evidence only nineteen times out of twenty. This would be especially true if the trial could lead to capital punishment. So we might examine the results of saying that beyond reasonable doubt means being right 99 times out of 100. The scientific term for this expression is a *confidence* of 99 percent.

To get this level of confidence we can allow one false identification for every 99 true cases. The prevalence of alcoholism in the general population of most of the common law countries is about 4 percent (physiological problems, above). So, to get 99 true cases we would normally need to study (100/4) × 99 people = 2,475 people. To be 99 percent certain of a correct identification of an alcoholic we can allow no more than one false identification for every 2,475 people in the general population. So we need a *specificity* of 99.96 percent. This value comes from the expression (2474/2475) × 100. The actual situation is not as bad as this since alcoholism in defendants and accused persons is probably much more prevalent than in the general population. Since we do not know exactly how prevalent, a prudent calculation is appropriate.

Let us suppose that 33.3 percent of the cases of child abuse involve alcohol abuse or dependence by the accused. To get 99 true cases we would need to study (100/33.3) × 99 people = 297 people. So here it would be ideal if we had a test that is (296/297) × 100, that is, 99.7 percent specific.

The tests used to identify alcoholics are not perfect, and the results of applying such tests can be discouraging unless seen in context. First on the list of discouraging news items is that practically none of the tests for alcoholism is anywhere near as specific as we would like. So there is a chance that individuals may be identified by the tests as alcoholics when they are not alcoholics. Second, most of the existing tests, or combinations of tests that could be modified to allow this level of specificity would likely lack so much *sensitivity* that they would be almost useless. Here, insensitive means that most cases of alcoholism would pass unnoticed.

What Are the Tests Going to Tell?

The tests in the following chapter may identify a person who has a significant problem with alcohol but the nature of the problem identified varies with the test. This may not be satisfactory for all purposes and, in particular, for the reader's purpose. This situation arises because of the state of the art and the variable nature of alcohol problems. Questioning the person under consideration is essential so that the true nature of the alcohol problem can be defined. We can never replace examination under oath with a series of tests administered in the abstract. Knowledge of the tests that follow may allow the reader to be in a better position to ask good questions. We leave the applicability of each test for the reader to decide, as much will depend on the circumstances. *The results of the tests provide clues, not answers.*

Four Meanings of "Outside the Normal Range"

The reader needs one last bit of information before proceeding with the rest of the book. From the subtitle above, you may guess that this is an area where scientists do not always mean what they say. It is useful to understand these meanings to appreciate expert testimony concerning normal values for a variety of quantitative results and not just for those concerning alcohol. So the authors give a little more information than is necessary for the purposes of this book.

Meaning One: The Literal Meaning

This meaning is easy to understand. Let's say that we obtain values of alcohol metabolic rates from a group of healthy subjects. The lowest value may be 12 mg/dL/hour and the highest value may be 20 mg/dL/hour. So any value obtained that is either below 12 or above 20 mg/dL/hour can be said to be outside the normal range (or reference range).

Meaning Two: Outside the Mean Plus or Minus Two Standard Deviations

This is not an uncommon meaning. The standard deviation (SD) measures the variability of a group of numbers. If you take the average (that is, the mean) and add twice the value of the standard deviation and subtract twice the value of the standard deviation you get a range. If the group under consideration is normal, the range of values is the normal range. Yet statistics tells us that the range defined in this manner covers only 95 percent of the values. What about the other 5 percent, are they not normal too? Yes, they are. *So a value may be inside the normal range using the first meaning but outside the normal range using the second meaning.* The following figure may aid understanding.

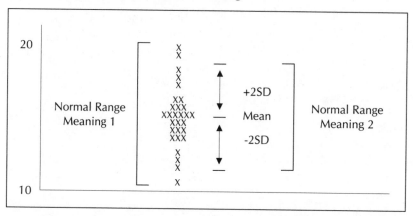

So the reader will not have a surprise in some future enterprise, we can note that it is not uncommon to use log-normal distributions. Here, the logarithm of each value is taken before the standard deviation is calculated. This is just a technique that allows the use of simple tests on complex data.

Meaning Three: Outside the Mean Plus or Minus Three Standard Deviations

The difference between this meaning and the last one is that ±3SD covers 99 percent of normal values.

Meaning Four: A Population-Qualified Meaning

The subjects in a normal population may be healthy but still not appropriate for the comparison at issue. Consider a normal range derived entirely from results obtained from male, Swedish, police cadets. It may or may not be an appropriate point of comparison for a sedentary, Japanese, middle-aged woman.

11
Tests for Alcoholism

Tests Based on Tolerance

Brain or Central Nervous System (CNS) Tolerance

Even an ordinary social drinker who consumes alcohol regularly will show some degree of tolerance to the effects of alcohol. With alcoholics, though, the degree of tolerance can be surprisingly large. People who work in the alcoholism field have had an intelligent conversation with an alcoholic and were later surprised to find that not only had he been drinking but at the time of the conversation the blood alcohol concentration was four times the legal limit. At the Addiction Research Foundation a few intoxicated patients have even walked out under their own steam with blood alcohol concentrations above 500 mg/dL. (Readers will kindly note that we don't put forward these records as a challenge. Also, the individuals concerned were actively discouraged from leaving the premises.)

The NCA Criteria

The National Council on Alcoholism of the United States says that if a person fulfills any of the following blood alcohol criteria then he is an alcoholic:

Alcohol concentration		
Blood (mg/dL) *or more*	*Breath (µg/dL)* *or more*	*Circumstance*
100	43	When visiting a physician.
150	65	Not obviously intoxicated.
300	130	At any time.

Approximately equivalent breath alcohol concentrations have been included for comparison.

These tests are mainly based on CNS tolerance. Presumably, the last criterion ("at any time") refers to voluntary consumption of alcohol with some knowledge of the likely consequences.

Values for the specificity and sensitivity of these tests are not easy to figure out. The reader may recall a mention in the last chapter that in the full NCA instrument there are ninety-one criteria. Also, the criteria committee noted that all the data must fit into a consistent whole to ensure a proper diagnosis. In this book we have used only major criteria that are likely to be answered in circumstances that may be of interest to the reader. Another problem is that brain damage may cause an alcoholic to lose tolerance despite continued heavy drinking.

Metabolic Tolerance

We saw earlier that some alcoholics metabolize alcohol faster than social drinkers. If we know the results of two blood or breath analyses then we can estimate the metabolic rate. We can then compare it with the ranges of values common for alcoholics and social drinkers to see into which group the subject will likely fall. (Note that this approach ignores the fact that the alcohol elimination profile is not linear.)

The Calculation. Let's say that a person has a blood alcohol concentration of 200 mg/dL and three hours later the concentration was down to 110 mg/dL. The metabolic rate is (200 − 110)/3 = 30 mg/dL/hour.

Problems in Getting the Data. To estimate a rate of decline of alcohol concentrations we require two or more data points. There are two problems that you may encounter. First, two or more tests were not administered. Second, the tests were so close in time that they are useless.

The common police practice of administering two breath tests fifteen minutes apart does not yield useful rates-of-decline results. In a period of fifteen minutes the alcohol concentration does not fall more than the error involved in the tests. We need an interval between the tests of at least a couple of hours to give a reasonable estimate of the rate of decline of alcohol concentrations.

A practice that would give more confidence to the result would be to take a measurement, say, every forty-five minutes for about four hours. This happens infrequently in busy police stations or in a busy hospital unless it is required for medical purposes. There is no reason, though, that a subject could not submit himself to such a test in a private laboratory if it was to his advantage to do so.

Acetate Concentration. There is a way of getting around the requirement of two or more samples. It turns out that the *concentration* of blood acetate (chapter 3) is proportional to the *rate* of alcohol disappearance. The concentration of acetate is somewhat independent of the concentration of alcohol while the alcohol concentration is above a low level. Finnish scientists have examined this phenomenon in elegant experiments and attempted to deploy it for identification.

The requirements of the test are:

1. The subject must have alcohol "on board" at the time of the test.
2. The subject must have enhanced alcohol metabolism at the time of the test.

A problem with this method is that most hospital and forensic laboratories do not analyze acetate as a matter of routine.

Specificity and Sensitivity. Whether metabolic rate is determined by two or more direct alcohol measurements or by measuring acetate concentration, the specificity and sensitivity are not high. When we define the normal range as the mean ± 2SD, we can expect incorrect identification of social drinkers as alcohol abusers (more than 80 grams/day) in about 10 percent of cases. The sensitivity of the test is only 65 percent. For these reasons it is best to conduct this type of test in conjunction with other tests.

Other Tests Based upon the Direct Measurement of Alcohol

Daily Morning Urine (or Other Fluid) Testing

This has been used in a six-month study at an alcoholic liver disease outpatient clinic at the Addiction Research Foundation. The presence of alcohol in a morning urine sample identifies either heavy drinking during the previous evening (probable alcohol abuse) or drinking during the morning (probable alcohol dependence). The analysis of alcohol in any other fluid could serve the same purpose.

The results of the study were interesting because less than a fifth of the patients admitted drinking every time they did. Also, patients with alcohol in these morning urine samples were very convincing in denying drinking most of the time.

There is the obvious problem that work of this nature cannot be done retrospectively. This technique is more useful for assessing the results of treatment (see chapter 12) than for identification of alcohol problems. Still, an isolated finding of alcohol in the body after a night's sleep may be objective evidence of significant alcohol problems.

The next two tests are of little importance for the purposes of identification. We make brief mention only for the sake of completeness.

Sweat Patch

A sweat-patch technique has only been tried in research studies. The patient wears a plastic-covered paper patch on his ankle covered by a plastic film. Scientists hoped that the alcohol excreted in sweat would remain in the patch until removal and analysis at weekly intervals. Unfortunately, the test does not work, because the alcohol back-diffuses through the skin into the blood and is lost.

Telephone Bugging

Yes, it *is* possible. A small alcohol sensor could be put into the mouthpiece of a telephone and inaudible signals corresponding to breath alcohol concentrations could be sent out over the telephone wires. The authors have a design for such a device. Though there are many politicians worth testing it on we have not yet found an opposition party willing to fund the work.

Questionnaires and Appearance

Detecting alcohol dependence from either the answers to questionnaires or from an individual's appearance is a science unto itself, but we shall consider some tests that are simple to use and may be useful. There are, though, some things that the reader should note:

1. The tests come from work with persons who had "asked" for help with their alcohol problems. The reader, on the other hand, may be faced with a situation in which the individual is trying to hide his problems. So the same results can hardly be expected.

2. It is not always certain what type of alcohol problem (abuse or dependence) is identified in the tests.

3. The consequences of alcohol problems depend, in part, on the length of time the problems have existed in the individual. So a new alcohol abuser may be more difficult to identify than an old one.

4. The first three questionnaires contain questions that are very direct and may be threatening to the subject.

5. Honest answers are required.

The One-Liner

The question is, "Do you have a problem with alcohol?" Readers will note that we have not specified the nature of the problem. Instead, the individual being questioned decides whether he has *any* problems with alcohol. Many of those with alcohol problems recognize them. Often, though, an alcoholic will deny that he has problems with alcohol and so more elaborate questions may be suitable. (Persons with alcohol-related problems often deny this aspect of reality. There may be many causes for the denial, but a common reason is that acceptance of the problem causes anxiety.)

The CAGE Questionnaire

The acronym *CAGE* comes from the key words in the four questions:

> Ever felt the need to **C** ut down drinking?
> > Ever felt **A** nnoyed by criticism of drinking?
> > Ever had **G** uilty feelings about drinking?
> Ever take a morning **E** ye opener?

This simple test was developed in North Carolina and has been validated in London and elsewhere.

Positive answers to three or four questions will identify persons with significant alcohol problems with a specificity of up to 100 percent. The sensitivity is 50 to 95 percent depending on the nature of the problem with alcohol.

Two positive answers may well give cause for concern but this is the point at which specificity starts to become a problem. So, two positive answers alone are not sufficient to determine alcohol abuse or dependence. Still, nonalcoholics rarely give positive answers to the second or fourth questions. Consequently, positive answers to either of these two questions should alert the interviewer.

Note that there are some patients who, although in residence in an alcohol rehabilitation facility and who give positive answers to all four questions, still deny that they have problems with alcohol.

The SAAST Questionnaire

The Self-Administered Alcohol Screening Test was developed at the Mayo Clinic in Minnesota and is a derivative of the Michigan Alcohol Screening Test (MAST). The original SAAST test has thirty-five questions but a shorter version consisting of nine items does a pretty good job of identifying alcoholics according to DSM-III criteria. The following questions have been altered slightly from the originals, mainly so that only positive responses are counted.

1. Do you feel that you drink more than average?
2. Do close relatives ever worry or complain about your drinking?
3. Are you sometimes unable to stop drinking when you want to?
4. Has your drinking ever created problems between you and your spouse or a near relative?
5. Do you ever drink in the morning?
6. Have you ever felt the need to cut down on your drinking?
7. Has a doctor ever told you to stop drinking?
8. If you have ever been a patient in a psychiatric ward of a hospital, was drinking part of the problem?
9. Have you ever been arrested because of driving while intoxicated?

A score of five or more yes answers identifies 90 percent of DSM-III alcoholics with a specificity of 99.4 percent. A score of four or more identifies 95 percent of DSM-III alcoholics with a specificity of 97.6 percent.

The Trauma Questionnaire

The trauma questionnaire is a test that identifies some persons who have been severely intoxicated at some point in their lives and suffered traumatic injuries as a result.

The possibility always exists that the alcohol-related injuries took place many years before and that the subject has been on the straight and narrow ever since. Of course, this leads to a conflict with the a priori moral pronouncement that an alcoholic is an alcoholic for life. But perhaps it is easy to agree that in most legal proceedings little or no account should be taken of a previous life-style, especially if the subject has long lost his dependence on alcohol and no longer abuses alcohol.

The trauma history questionnaire consists of five questions.

Since your eighteenth birthday, have you:

1. Had any fractures or dislocations to your bones or joints?
2. Been injured in a road traffic accident?
3. Had an injury to your head?
4. Been injured in an assault or fight (excluding sports)?
5. Been injured after drinking?

This questionnaire was evaluated in a study of social drinkers and alcohol abusers who were seeking help for their problems. The average alcohol abuser who sought help for his problems had a score of three whereas the average social drinker had a score of one.

The problems in application of this test are the somewhat poor sensitivity and specificity. Some alcohol abusers have a score of zero, and it is easy to see how a social drinker can get a score of three. Still, a score of two or more *suggests* that there is an alcohol abuse problem.

Alcoholism in the Family

There are genetic and home environmental components to alcoholism, but most children of alcoholics do not become alcoholics. Thus, questions concerning alcoholism of the parents cannot give unambiguous identification of alcoholics. Still, a positive family history should alert the interviewer.

Parent/Child. A family history of alcoholism increases the risk of alcoholism in the children. A third of alcoholics have at least one alcoholic parent. However, the relationship between alcoholic mother and daughter is far weaker than that between alcoholic father and son.

Twins. If one identical twin is an alcoholic then there is about a 50 percent chance that the other twin is also an alcoholic. With fraternal twins the concordance is less and of little predictive value.

Personality Tests

There are personality tests that can detect alcoholism and the Minnesota Multiphasic Personality Inventory (MMPI) test is a well-known example. The problems with these tests are that they consist of hundreds of questions and they require experts for interpretation. One advantage is that these measures do not usually contain questions that refer directly to drinking behavior.

Appearance

The elements of a test based on a person's appearance have been abstracted from a checklist for a proposed clinical examination in the detection of alcohol problems. The elements that require medical training and those that are unlikely to be attempted by the reader have been deleted along with the gradations used. Because of these changes, the test cannot be as specific and sensitive as the original.

The study was done on a group of people that consumed more than thirty drinks a week for eight years and reported a range of consequences related to drinking. They were compared with a group of social drinkers (six or fewer drinks per week and no more than two drinks per occasion).

Clinical sign	Times more commonly observed in alcoholics
Enlarged nose	4
Facial red skin	3
Skin "nicotine" stains	18
Red palms	4
Bruises, abrasions	6
Scars (nonsurgical)	2
Tattoos	5
Cigarette burns	*
Hand tremor	**

 * Seen in one in four of this group of alcoholics
   but in none of the social drinkers.
** Typically increased above normal

Several positive signs may suggest alcohol abuse but values of sensitivity and specificity cannot be offered.

Death Certificates

A death certificate might possibly record or suggest that alcohol abuse or dependence was associated with the cause of death. Similarly, a death certificate might record that alcoholic liver disease, or other alcohol-related disorder, was either the cause of death or was related to the cause of death. Usually though, these things of interest are not noted. If alcoholic liver disease was the cause of death and it is not recorded then it is most unlikely that brain damage would be recorded. It is even more unlikely that simple alcohol dependence would be noted. Anyhow, most alcoholics do not develop liver disease or brain damage.

There are various reasons why alcohol-related diseases and disorders are not recorded. For example, the person may be recorded as having died of a medical complication of alcoholic liver disease. Other reasons include that the proximate cause of death may have been accidental, or death may have been from natural causes.

A death certificate is only useful, for the present purposes, on those rare occasions when alcohol is mentioned. Otherwise, all that can be done is to question if the stated cause of death is consistent with the existence of alcohol problems.

Frequency of Changing Jobs

Job efficiency and performance are often poor in persons with alcohol-related problems (notable exceptions include Sir Winston Churchill). There is a greater incidence of absenteeism and accidents. There is also, on average, a reduction in reaction time, motivation, judgment, and the ability to handle stress. Because of the problems, these persons change jobs more frequently than most others. And because of the denial phenomenon, they often have the belief that the stress is caused more by the job than by the drinking. There are, though, many possible reasons for changing jobs and not changing jobs. So for our purposes, the frequency of employment changes would be such a nonspecific test that it would be useless.

Other Blood Tests for Alcoholism

Many tests are being developed and examined in research laboratories. The idea is to develop objective tests that do not depend on the cooperation of the subject (apart from obtaining the sample). Although much of the published work shows skill and imagination in the approaches, with one exception the results show that nature is guarding its secrets jealously. In the following sections we describe a few tests that are well known, potentially useful, or interesting.

Mean Corpuscular Volume (MCV) and Serum Gamma-Glutamyl Transpeptidase (GGT)

Mean corpuscular volume (MCV) refers to the volume of the red blood cells, and serum gamma-glutamyl transpeptidase (GGT) is an enzyme that circulates in the blood. They are commonly measured in hospital laboratories. Heavy consumption of alcohol (about five drinks or more per day) frequently causes abnormal results to be obtained in 75 percent of alcoholic patients. Unfortunately, abnormal results on these tests can be caused by a variety of illnesses. So the specificity of these tests either alone or in combination is insufficient for identification.

The tests can be useful when they are used on the same person at different times. A decrease in GGT concentration over a period of several months, for example, may show that the patient has got his drinking under control. This may be especially true if the GGT concentration was outside the normal range to begin with.

Carbohydrate-deficient Transferrin (CDT)

As of July 1990, there is no doubt that the best-looking blood (actually serum) test for alcoholism comes from Sweden. It involves the measurement of carbohydrate-deficient transferrin (CDT) and the results are very promising.

In a large study, the Swedish authors found a sensitivity of 91 percent in identifying alcoholics (defined as persons consuming more than sixty grams of alcohol per day) with a specificity of 99 percent. (And even this figure of 99 percent may be considered low as the persons incorrectly identified were female hospital patients over the age of eighty years, that is, patients in whom a few abnormal results may not be unexpected.) In a more recent, though smaller study, of this test by other investigators the results showed a sensitivity of 87 percent and a specificity of 100 percent.

A patent for the test has been issued in Sweden, and presumably the Pharmacia Company will soon be selling a kit for this laboratory measurement.

Tests Based on Metabolic Interference

We saw earlier that alcohol usually reduces the metabolism of other compounds. If these other compounds are naturally present in the body or are present in alcoholic beverages, then heavy alcohol consumption will cause an increase in the concentrations. Finnish scientists have been notable in recent contributions to this field. They have studied methanol, which is present in small quantities even in legal alcoholic beverages and is produced naturally in the body in low concentrations. They have also studied naturally produced compounds called dolichols.

Although the tests give results that are of scientific interest, they do not, by themselves, give unambiguous identification of alcoholics. When we define the normal range as the mean ±2SD, we can expect incorrect identification of social drinkers as alcohol abusers in about 5 percent of cases. The sensitivity of the test is 68 percent. So these tests would have to be used with others for good methods of identification.

ID: Computer Program for the Identification of Alcohol Abuse/Dependence

To obtain the ID program follow the instructions given in the section "A Note on the Companion Computer Programs," following appendix 2.

The program is a computerized checklist of the tests given in this chapter. After answering the questions, the program gives a listing of the indicators of alcohol abuse/dependence.

Please note that the tests are generally independent. There is, therefore, no way to give a cumulative probability that a subject has alcohol problems. Positive responses should be viewed as clues to the existence of the problems. The greater the number of clues the greater is the probability that such problems exist. In as far as it has been possible, the weight that should be attached to individual clues is discussed above. We suggest that it may be useful to first try out the program on friends and colleagues whose drinking is not problematic. In this way, unusual patterns of responses will be more readily discerned when they occur.

12
Court-Ordered Treatment of Alcoholism

THERE IS NO such thing as a hopeless alcohol abuser or a hope-less alcoholic. Admittedly, the treatment of some persons is difficult and it may need to be lengthy, but everyone who has a problem with alcohol can be treated.

Often a court will specify that a convicted person must undergo treatment for alcoholism. If this is the extent of the order then we have no objection to it. The court can leave the problems of treatment to those who are best able to consider them. On those rare occasions when the court specifies a particular type of treatment, then there may be cause for concern. The questions that should always arise are:

1. What type of alcohol problem does the person have?

2. What type of treatment is being recommended?

3. What type of treatment facility is being recommended?

4. What is the desired result—moderation or abstinence?

5. How does one measure the desired result?

What follows is a very brief account of the modern approach to treatment and the ways of assessing it.

Distinguishing Alcohol Abuse and Alcohol Dependence

As mentioned previously, alcohol abusers (problem drinkers) are the persons who have any of the variety of social and medical problems that go with heavy alcohol consumption but who are not dependent on the drug. The distinguishing features of persons suffering alcohol dependence are a yearning for the drug, tolerance to its effects, and withdrawal symptoms when they stop drinking. These features markedly reduce the ability of the subject to exercise restraint over his drinking behavior.

Although the definitions above are clear enough, in practice it is sometimes difficult to classify persons according to this scheme. One reason for this is that the longer that problems with alcohol persist the more severe the social and medical problems become. Eventually it becomes impossible to distinguish abuse from dependence. Another occasion when it is difficult to distinguish between these two categories is when a person moves back and forth between them.

The Category Determines the Treatment

The approaches to treatment are dictated by the nature of the problems.

Alcohol Abuse

The use of one or more of the following components has proven to be effective in treating alcohol abusers so that alcohol-related problems may be reduced:

admonishment

advice

brief counseling

education

social ostracism

training

help in the management of any other contemporaneous difficulties

Alcohol Dependence

Persons who are dependent on alcohol may require different measures. The variety of treatments include

drug treatment

group and family therapies

long-term counseling

psychotherapy

help in the management of any other contemporaneous difficulties

use of the principles of Alcoholics Anonymous.

Treatment may be given on an inpatient or on an outpatient basis depending on all the individual circumstances including the extent of the dependence.

Assessment of the Results of Treatment

Three methods are in common use to assess alcohol consumption:

1. The patient may give a valuable appraisal of the treatment. On the other hand, this view may be highly unreliable.

2. Persons who know the patient may give their opinion on the efficacy of the strategy. These persons may include the spouse or other family members, friends, colleagues, supervisor, physician, probation officer, and religious minister. Again, the appraisal may be valuable or unreliable.

3. An objective assessment of alcohol consumption may be obtained from the results of body fluid analyses. Naturally, these tests cost money, and there are not many facilities available to do the tests and interpret the results. There are even fewer facilities equipped to conduct research in the area.

Appendix 1
Conversion Tables

Conversion of Weights

From	To	Multiply by
Pounds	kilograms	0.454
Stones	kilograms	6.35

Conversion of volumes

From	To	Multiply by
Fl oz (U.K.)	milliliters	28.4
Fl oz (U.S.)	milliliters	29.6
Gills (U.K.)	milliliters	142
Gills (U.S.)	milliliters	118
Pints (U.K.)	milliliters	568
Pints (U.S.)	milliliters	473

Conversion of lengths

From	To	Multiply by
Inches	centimeters	2.54
Feet	centimeters	30.48

Conversion of molar alcohol units

From	To	Divide by
Millimolar	mg/dL	46

Appendix 2
Glasgow Coma Scale

EYES	Open	Spontaneously	4
		To verbal command	3
		To pain	2
	No response		1
BEST MOTOR RESPONSE	To verbal command	Obeys	6
	To painful stimulus	Localizes pain	5
		Flexion-withdrawal	4
		Flexion - abnormal (decorticate rigidity)	3
		Extension (decerebrate rigidity)	2
		No response	1
BEST VERBAL RESPONSE		Oriented and converses	5
		Disoriented and converses	4
		Inappropriate words	3
		Incomprehensible sounds	2
		No response	1
TOTAL			3–15

A Note on the Companion Computer Programs

G WYNNE GILES and Sue Sandrin wrote these computer programs for use by people who have no knowledge of computers and little knowledge of alcohol, so don't be afraid of them.

Although this book will stand alone, the use of the computer programs helps in understanding the ideas. The programs also allow you to make estimations that would otherwise be difficult or impossible. They let you ask the multitude of "but what if" questions that arise in professional work.

The programs that are available to use with this book are RISK, ID, and BBAC. RISK deals with estimating the risk of a traffic accident. ID deals with the identification of alcoholics. BBAC is an abbreviation for Blood and Breath Alcohol Concentrations. This program is concerned with the disposition of alcohol in the body. It is likely to be the program that you use most and from which you will get the most enjoyment. Various comparisons (for example, male versus female; with food versus without food) are made for you, and the program allows you to make your own comparisons. You also can examine the disposition of alcohol in the body after as many drinks as you care to put into the program (up to fifty). Blood and breath alcohol concentrations are calculated and plotted on a graph at intervals corresponding to every five minutes over the period that interests you. (More details on the programs are in the text at the appropriate places.)

What Kind of Computer Is Needed?

For RISK and ID, you just need an IBM-compatible personal computer. For BBAC this computer also must have graphics capability. A CGA or EGA or Hercules system or equivalent is sufficient. If you are not sure of what you have but know that you have a modern machine then you should have no difficulties.

Installing the Programs

There is nothing to install. The programs are ready to run off the diskettes. In fact, this is the only way that they will run.

Starting the Programs

If you have a hard disk in your computer and the program is on a floppy diskette:

1. Switch on the computer and wait for it to finish whatever it does when it first starts
2. Put the diskette in drive A
3. Type *A*: that is, type the letter *A* and then type a colon
4. Press the *ENTER* key
5. The computer should then print A:\> on the screen
6 Type the name of the program, for example, *RISK*
7. Press the *ENTER* key

If you don't have a hard disk you first have to load the DOS. Then you go to point 2 above.

To order the programs

Send a check or money order to:

> Dr. H.G. Giles
> Department of Pharmacology
> Medical Sciences Building
> University of Toronto
> Toronto, Ontario
> M5S 1A8
> Canada

Make check or money order payable to Dr. H.G. Giles

Please send me _____ copies of ID at $5 US each

_____ copies of RISK at $20 US each

_____ copies of BBAC at $95 US each

Canadian residents add appropriate taxes.

Specify _____5 1/4 inch or _____3 1/2 inch diskette

Name _____

Address _____

_____

_____

_____

_____

Index

Absorption, 9–12, 29–30, 45
Acetaldehyde, 23, 47–49
Acetate, 23, 47, 105–106
Accuracy, 59–60
ADH, 23, 47, 57
Age, advanced, 67–68
Age and body water, 12–13
Alcohol abuser, 97, 118
Alcohol dehydrogenase, 23, 47, 57
Aldehyde dehydrogenase, 23, 26, 47, 49
ALDH, 23, 26, 47, 49
Antabuse, 47–48
Aqueous humor, 62
Assessment of treatment, 119–120

Back-calculation, 28–34
Barbiturates, 47
Beverages, 2, 11, 88–91
Biotransformation, 9
Blindness, 1, 4, 46
Blood samples, 14, 55–57
Blood serum, 15–16
Blood plasma, 14–16
Blood:breath ratio, 66–70
Body fluids, 15
Body size, 12–14, 51
Body water, 12–14, 51–53
Brain damage, 39–41
Brain tolerance, 25, 36–37, 41–42, 78, 103–104
Breast milk, 12, 18–19, 34
Breath, 16–17, 34, 58–59, 62–70
Breath freshening sprays, 8

CAGE questionnaire, 108
Calcium carbimide, 47–48
Calories, 41

Cancer, 43
Capacity, mental, 41–42
Carbohydrate-deficient transferrin, 114
CDT, 114
Central nervous system, 25, 39, 41–42, 103–104
Cerebrospinal fluid, 74
Characteristics of alcohol, 1
Chloral hydrate, 46
Chlorpropamide, 49
Chromatography, gas, 58, 60
Chronic obstructive pulmonary disease, 68
Cirrhosis, 42, 96
CNS tolerance, 25, 36–37, 41–42, 103–104
Colds, 67
Concentration of alcoholic beverages, 3–4, 88–91
Concentration units, 2–3, 17
Confidence, 99
Contraceptives, oral, 53
Conversion to metric units, 4, 13, 121
Convulsions, 40
Cosmetics, 7–8
Cyclosporine, 7

Death, samples obtained after, 61–62
Death certificates, 112–113
Delirium tremens, 40
Denatured alcohol, 1
Density, 1, 6
Distribution, 12–16, 29
Disulfiram, 47–48
Dolichols, 115
DSM-III, 96, 109
DT's, 40

Employment problems, 113
Endogenous alcohol, 26–27
Error: in breath analysis, 58–59, 65–70; instrument in, 59–61; in preserving a sample, 56–57, 58–59; reporting, 16; in taking a blood sample, 55–56; in transposition from breath to blood, 62–70; in transposition from urine to blood, 70–72
Excretion, 9, 34

FAE, 43–44, 54
Family, 110–111
FAS, 43–44, 54
Feminization, 38–39
Fetal alcohol effects, 43, 54
Fetal alcohol syndrome, 43–44, 54
Flusher, 26
Food, 10
Food flavoring agents, 8

Gargling solutions, 8
Gamma-glutamyltranspeptidase, 113–114
Gender neutralization, 38
GGT, 113–114
Gout, 39

Heart, 44
Hepatitis, 42
Hepatomegaly, 42

Illicitly produced beverages, 3–4
Immune system, 43
Injuries, traumatic, 25, 77–80
Intoxication, 41
Isopropanol, 1, 55, 56

Jobs, changing, 113

Lachrymal fluid, 15, 74
Last gulp defense, 12, 73
Liver, 9–10, 25, 42

MAST questionnaire, 109
MCV, 113–114
Mean corpuscular volume, 113–114

Menstrual cycle, 53
Mental incapacity, 41–42
Metabolic interference, 114–115
Metabolic tolerance, 24–25, 104–106
Metabolism, 9, 23–24, 45–47
Methanol, 1, 46
Methyl alcohol, 1, 46
Metronidazole, 49
Mickey Finn, 46
Milk, breast, 12, 18–19, 34
Miscarriage, 54
Molar, 17, 121
Mole, 17, 121
Moonshine, 3–4
Mouth wash, 8

Names, 1
National Council on Alcoholism, criteria of alcoholism, 97, 103–104
NCA criteria of alcoholism, 97, 103–104
Neonate, 19, 43–44
Normal range, 100–102
Nutrition, 26, 41

Oral contraceptives, 53
Orientals, 26
Origin, 1

Pancreas, 44
Parents, 110–111
Partial sample defense, 68
Peripheral nutritis, 41
Personality tests, 111
Phenytoin, 47
Physical activity, 10
Physiological problems, 96
Plasma, 14–16
Police policy, 69–70
Post mortem samples, 61–62
Poteen, 3–4
Potheen, 3–4
Precision, 59–60
Preservation of samples, 56–57
Problem drinker, 97, 118–119
Proof units, 2–3
Psychiatric definition, 96
Pulmonary disease, 68

Ratio, blood:breath, 66–70
Ratio, urine:blood, 70–73
Red blood cells, 15, 44
Regurgitation, 68–69

SAAST questionnaire, 109
Saliva, 12, 15, 34, 74
SD, 101
Sensitivity, 105–106, 108, 112, 114
Serum, 15
Small intestine, 9, 10
Smoking, 43, 47, 67
Social drinker, 98
Sociological problems, 95–97
Specificity, 60, 105–106, 108, 109,
    112, 114
Sperm defects, 44
Standard deviation, 101
Stomach, 9–11, 61–62
Stomach contents, 61
Stomach removal, 11
Sweat patch, 106–107

Tears, 15, 34
Telephone bugging, 107
Temposil, 47–48
Tolbutamide, 49
Tolerance, brain, 25, 36–37, 41–42,
    78, 103–104

Tolerance, CNS, 25, 36–37, 41–42, 78,
    103–104
Tolerance, metabolic, 24, 25, 104–106
Total body water, 12–14, 51–53
Transposition errors, 62–70, 70–72
Trauma questionnaire, 109–110
Treatment of alcoholism, 117–120
Tremor, 40, 112
Twins, 111

Unit system for alcoholic drinks, 7
Units of concentration, 2–3, 17
Urine, 12, 15, 70–73
Urine:blood ratio, 70–73
Uses of alcohol, 1

Volume of a drink, 4–5

Water, total body, 12–14, 51–53
Water content of body liquids, 15–16
Weight of alcohol in a drink, 6–7
Wernicke's syndrome, 41
Withdrawal, 39–41
Women, 51–54
World Health Organiztion,
    alcoholism definition, 96

About the Authors

Gwynne Giles, B.Sc., LL.B., M.S., Ph.D. studied science and law in Wales, England, the United States, and Canada. He is a scientist at the Addiction Research Foundation and an assistant professor of pharmacology at the University of Toronto.

Bhushan Kapur, B.Sc., D. Phil., studied in India and Switzerland. He is director of the clinical laboratory at the Addiction Research Foundation and an assistant professor of clinical biochemistry at the University of Toronto.

Both authors have published widely and appear in court as expert witnesses.